CLINICAL CARDIOLOGY AND EXAMINATION

CLINICAL CARDIOLOGY AND EXAMINATION

Dr. Rajesh S. Roy

MD Internal Medicine
Fellowship in Basic Echocardiography
Fellowship in Advanced Echocardiography
Fellowship in TEE, 2D Strain, 3D Echocardiography
Certificate Course in Diabetes and Cardiac Care

Senior Consultant and Associate Professor,
Department of Medicine,
Parul Institute of Medical Sciences and Research, Baroda.

Co-ordinator and Chief Echo cardiologist,
Department of Non-invasive Cardiology,
Parul Institute of Medical Sciences and Research, Baroda.

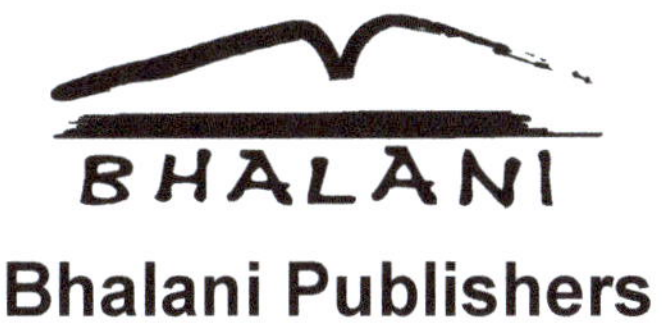

Bhalani Publishers

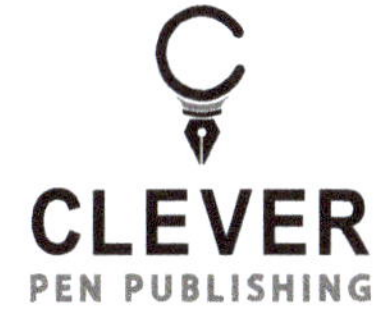

First Edition: 2021

Published by:

BHALANI PUBLISHERS and
Clever Pen Publishing
(A joint venture between Bhalani Publishers and National Medical Book House)
D-2 Neelkanth Business Park Co-op. Premises Society Lt.
Nathani Road
Vidyavihar (West)
Mumbai 400086
Mob.: 09867214519

Email:
bhalanipublishers@gmail.com
cleverpen9@gmail.com

ISBN 978-93-83794-08-9

Printed & Bound in India

This Book is Dedicated

to

My parents, Mr. Sukumar K. Roy and Mrs. Kusum S. Roy,

who even with limited resources and money,

made me what I am today.

My wife Dr. Jyotika Patel Roy,

who has always been my power and support and

because of whom I could concentrate solely on

making this book.

And lastly my Teachers

who made me capable of writing this book, especially

Dr. Rakesh Gupta Sir

whom I consider as my idol and mentor

Foreword

Dr. Rajesh Roy, Associate Professor, Department of Medicine; Co-ordinator and Chief Echo cardiologist, Department of Non-Invasive Cardiology, Parul Institute of Medical Sciences and Research, Vadodara, happens to be one of my brightest students. His clinical acumen, hard work, and devout nature impressed one and all. His immediate affirmative response to any assignment was very well recognized in the whole of the department.

Clinical signs play a significant role in the diagnosis of a patient suffering from cardiovascular disease. An understanding of the basics of clinical cardiology in the form of inspection, palpation, auscultation, and percussion plays an imperative role in the proper diagnosis. A very good attempt has been made by Dr. Rajesh Roy, in making you understand the various aspects of these important signs by compiling them into a single manuscript, as done previously by " Hutchinson". The present manuscript will be a boon to budding physicians in understanding the basics of medicine and cardiology.

I wish him all success in this venture with the hope that censorious acclaim by the various expert will lead to the publication of the next breed of this manual very soon.

Dr. Rakesh Gupta

MD, FASE, FISCU, FACC (USA), FCSI, FIAE, FICP, FIMSA, FIACTA (INDIA)

Formerly Cardiologist

Thomas Jefferson University Hospital, Philadelphia, USA

Director and Chief Cardiologist

JROP Institute of Echocardiography, Ultrasound & Vascular Doppler, Delhi, India
JROP Healthcare, C-1/16, Ashok Vihar - II, Delhi - 110052, India
Vice President: Cardiological Society of India (2016-2017) (2018-2020)

Chairman

Accreditation & Fellowship committee of IAE (2002 to present)
Past President: Cardiological Society of India (Delhi Branch 2012-2014)
Past Associate Editor: Indian Heart Journal of CSI (2006-2010)

Past Editor in Chief

Journal of Indian Academy of Echocardiography (2012-2016)

Past President

Indian Academy of Echocardiography (2006-2008)

Governing Council Member

Indian College of Physicians of API (2015-2017)
Email: rakeshecho@gmail.com, jrop2001@yahoo.com
www.jrop.in, www.echocourse.in, www.echocentre.in

Preface

It has probably been since my UG days that I felt the need of a book in cardiology that should have been a bit simple and concise but at the same time with good explanations too.

This book "Clinical Cardiology and Examination" has been written by me with the hope that it would help everyone in understanding the basic concepts of cardiology.

I went through several good books and Journals and tried to compile the information and knowledge at one place with simplified language.

This book has 17 chapters pertaining to some basic, but very important topics in cardiology like General examination, Inspection, Palpation, Percussion, Auscultation, Blood pressure, Arterial pulse, JVP, Heart sounds, and Murmurs.

This book has been made keeping in mind not only Undergraduates and Postgraduates, but also practicing clinicians who would find this book useful in refreshing their skills that they might have read quite long ago.

Truly speaking, I have tried my level best to write as simple as possible and have tried to draw very neat and clear figures. I am thankful to Parul University (where I work), Dr. Rajesh U Patel, Dr. Som Lakhani, Dr. Sriranga R, and Dr. Chetan Chauhan for providing me with some very good patient photographs.

I would also like to thank Mr. Rajesh Bhalani and Mr. Rushabh Bhalani from Bhalani Publishers for showing their belief in me and motivating me constantly.

However, I would also like to say that this is my first attempt to write a book and I accept that there may be some errors.

But I promise that I will try to rectify them as the time passes and will try to come up with new literature, concepts, ideas and good figures.

I request the readers to give their valuable feedback on this book at rajeshroy2255@gmail.com so that I can come up with even better versions of this book in future.

Thanking everyone
Dr. Rajesh S. Roy

Contents

Feedback

Help Us Improve

Scan the QR code
and give your feedback
Or
You can email us your feedback on

- ☞ bhalanipublishers@gmail.com
- ☞ cleverpen9@gmail.com

CHAPTER 1 History and Examination of CVS

HISTORY TAKING AND SYMPTOMATOLOGY IN CARDIOLOGY

- The importance of history taking in cardiology can never be underestimated as rightly said by Sir William Osler (Father of Modern Medicine) ----"Listen to your patient, he is telling you the diagnosis".
- A good clinical history and a proper physical examination remains the mainstay of a proper therapeutic approach to any patient suspicious of having a cardiovascular disease.
- It not only reduces much of the fear and anxiety of the patient and helps build a proper rapport with the clinician, but also avoids unnecessary tests and investigations and saves the patient's money.
- Many times elaborating the history from the relatives and friends of the patient is helpful in knowing the course and seriousness of the illness and also helps in explaining the prognosis to them which avoids any future medicolegal issues which is very common these days.
- One may even make his own checklist for history taking, if required which would avoid missing any relevant point(s).
- In day to day practice, a cardiac patient may come to you for cardiac symptoms like dyspnea, chest pain or dizziness (syncope) or some general practitioner might refer him to you after finding some abnormal findings like a murmur or abnormal investigations like an abnormal ECG or X-Ray.
- There is no term like "IMPOSSIBLE" in medical science. Hence we should always remember that even Fever can occur as a symptom of cardiac origin e.g, Atrial myxoma, Infective endocarditis, Perivalvular abscess, etc.
- Orthopnea and Paroxysmal nocturnal dyspnea (PND) should give you a hint about the presence of raised left atrial pressure (LAP).

PAROXYSMAL NOCTURNAL DYSPNEA (PND)

⇨ Breathlessness occurs 2 to 3 hours after sleep and relieved after sitting for 10 to 20 minutes.

⇨ There is ↑LAP due to interstitial and intra-alveolar edema.

⇨ MC cause of PND is Mitral stenosis (MS).

- Conditions mimicking PND are obesity, nocturnal asthma, anxiety, frequent pulmonary embolism, post nasal drip.

ORTHOPNEA

- Breathlessness in supine posture which is relieved immediately on sitting.
- Occurs due to ↑ venous return leading to pulmonary congestion.
- Causes include LVF (MC), COPD, ascites.
- PND patients fall in NYHA grade III, and Orthopnea patients fall in NYHA grade IV.

PLATYPNEA

- Breathlessness in sitting or upright posture which is relieved by lying supine.
- Characteristically seen in LA myxoma.

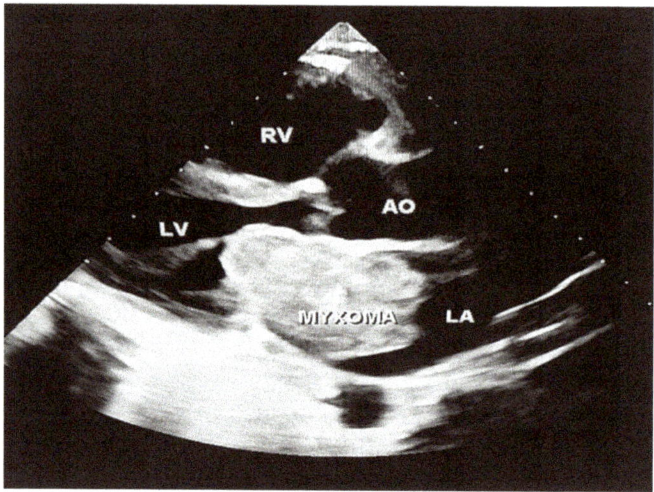

Fig. 1.1: A large LA myxoma.

TREPOPNEA

- Breathlessness in lateral posture.
- Seen with LA myxoma obstructing the mitral valve (MV) in lateral posture.

Breathlessness/Dyspnea in the resting state

- Functional state
- PE
- Pulmonary edema
- Pneumothorax

Sudden breathlessness

⇨ Foreign body lodgement in the airways
⇨ PE
⇨ Tension pneumothorax
⇨ Sudden onset pulmonary edema

Drugs precipitating breathlessness

⇨ Beta blockers (by causing bronchoconstriction)
⇨ Digoxin, if given in HOCM
⇨ Steroids

Cardiovascular causes of breathlessness

⇨ CCF
⇨ Cardiomyopathies
⇨ Valve abnormalities
⇨ Congenital heart diseases (CHD)
⇨ Pericardial abnormalities

However, it is very important to understand that dyspnea can present along with other symptoms as well to give us the hint about the disease like:

⇨ **Dyspnea + Fever:** TB pericarditis, viral myocarditis, and some non cardiac causes like pneumonia, pleuritis, lung cancers.
⇨ **Dyspnea + Cyanosis:** CHD and COPD.
⇨ **Dyspnea + Chest pain:** Acute coronary syndrome, pericarditis, COPD, tension pneumothorax.
⇨ **Dyspnea + Pedal edema:** CCF, Constrictive pericarditis, massive pleural effusion.

- One classification to assess the severity of dyspnea of cardiac origin is The New York Heart Association (NYHA) classification of dyspnea.

NYHA CLASSIFICATION→→

Class I- Dyspnea only on severe exertion

Class II-Dyspnea on ordinary activities

Class III-Dyspnea at less than ordinary activities

Class IV-Dyspnea even at rest.

- Generalized weakness can occur due to chronic low cardiac output e.g., chronic ischemia, inflow obstruction, pulmonary hypertension, cardiomyopathies, etc.

- Swelling of the feet (peripheral edema) is most of the times seen as a cardiac symptom like in CCF , Tricuspid Regurgitation, Constrictive pericarditis (CP), etc.
- But one should not forget that peripheral edema may occur in renal disease also wherein the edema is more in the morning in association with periorbital edema and tends to decrease as the day progresses with/without a reduced urine output.
- Pedal edema of hepatic origin (hypoalbuminemia) may be associated with ascites, persisting throughout the day and with/without a history of alcoholism.
- However in edema of cardiac origin, we must expect a raised Jugular venous pressure.
- One of the cardinal cardiac symptoms for which patients come to the cardiac department is chest pain.
- A classic "cardiac chest pain" is described as tightness, squeezing, heaviness or burning sensation, located mostly in the retro sternal region and may be radiating to the ulnar border of the left hand, shoulders, jaw or neck with /without dyspnea and perspiration.
- The gesture of the patient is also important as usually a patient of acute coronary syndrome would hold his clenched fist in front of his chest while describing the chest pain......."Levine's sign".

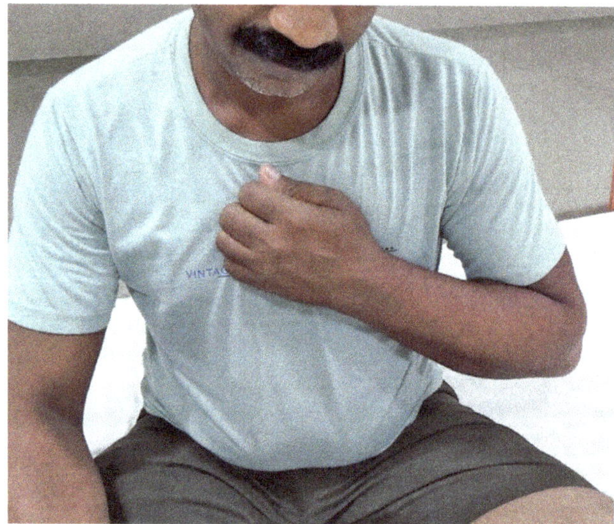

Fig. 1.2: Levine's sign.

- Chest pain which can be pinpointed by a finger, located near the left mammary area or going below the umbilicus is usually non cardiac in origin.
- A proper history about the onset and duration of the chest pain can help us differentiate Acute coronary syndrome (pain duration ≥ 20 minutes) from Unstable angina (UA) or Prinzmetal's angina (unprovoked at rest) or from angina pectoris which lasts for 2 to 5 minutes. The pain may get relieved by taking nitrates in angina pectoris, but if it remains even longer than 10 to 15 minutes then think of UA or MI or some non cardiac causes.

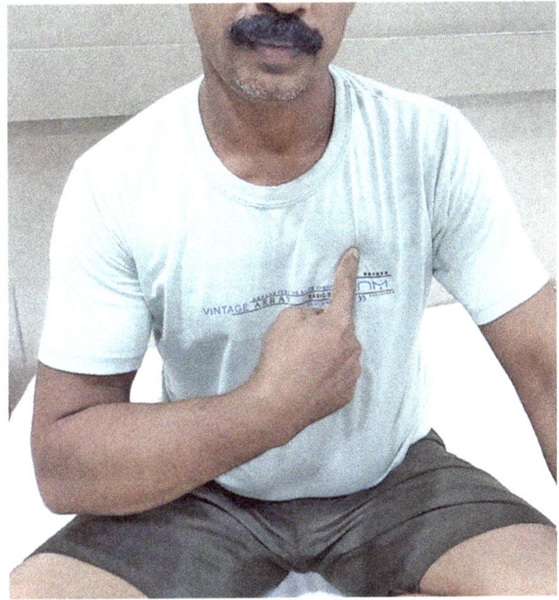

Fig. 1.3: Chest pain pin-pointed to the left mammary area is usually non-cardiac in origin.

- Chest pain in supine position and more in the trapezius region and relieved by sitting upright and leaning forward suggests a diagnosis of acute pericarditis.
- Pain of aortic dissection is classically a sudden onset tearing or crushing pain at the central back, sometimes radiating to the lower limbs or abdomen in cases of descending aorta involvement, while pain in the neck, jaw, throat, or face indicates ascending aorta involvement. One must also pay attention to see for features of Marfan's syndrome and h/o trauma, either direct or iatrogenic.

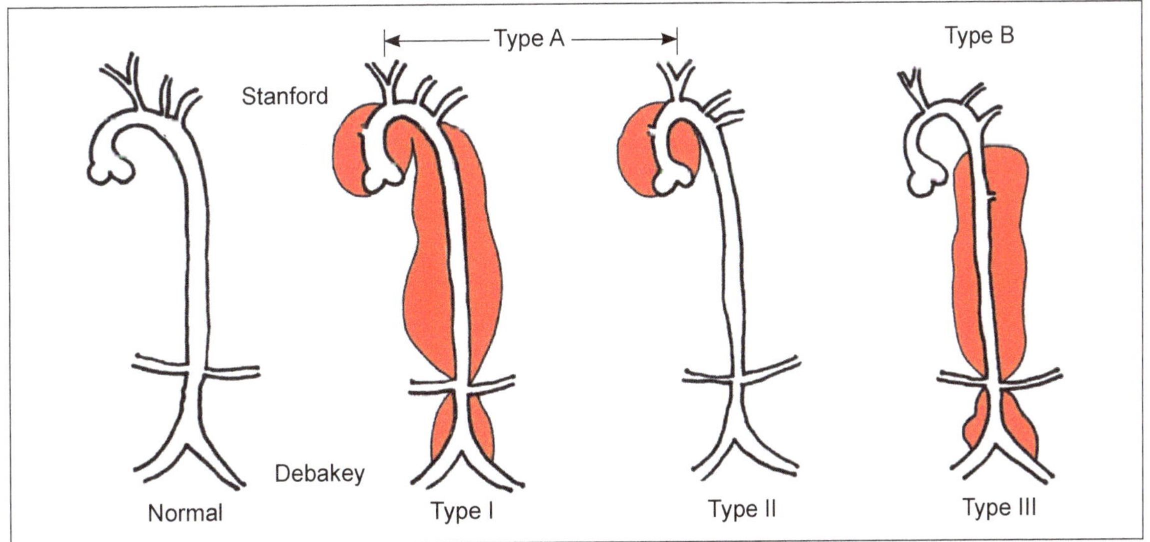

Fig. 1.4: Aortic dissection with Debakey and Stanford classifications.

- Severe aortic stenosis (AS) can cause chest pain (angina) with dyspnea and syncope.
- Chest pain in mitral valve prolapse (MVP) is spontaneous in onset, not related to exercise and is because of papillary muscle stretching.

Non cardiac causes of chest pain includes

⇨ GIT: Peptic ulcer disease, esophageal spasm, GERD, pancreatitis, gallbladder diseases.

⇨ Pulmonary: Pneumonia, pneumothorax, PE.

⇨ Musculoskeletal: Costochondritis(Tietze syndrome), myalgias, cervical spondylosis.

⇨ Neurogenic: Herpes zoster.

⇨ Functional: Psychiatric illnesses like depression, anxiety, psychosis.

- Sometimes however, the patient complains of symptoms other than chest pain, but cardiac in origin. These symptoms are called Anginal Equivalents.
- Anginal Equivalents include symptoms like dizziness, belching, fatigue, and syncope.

Importance of age in cardiovascular system(some examples)

⇨ Angina classically affects males > 50 years of age and females > 60 years of age.

⇨ A cardiac murmur developing after 6months of age is never due to VSD.

⇨ Juvenile MS occurs before 17 years of age.

⇨ Aortic valve calcification is common after 40 years of age.

⇨ Mortality risk of open cardiac surgery after 80 years of age is around 25%.

⇨ CABG benefits ↑after 50 years of age but ↓if the age is > 75 years.

Hence, proper age and its correlation to CVS is very important in history taking.

Importance of sex in cardiovascular system

⇨ CAD occurs about 10 years late in females compared to males.

⇨ CAD is not common before menopause.

Importance of drug history in cardiovascular system

⇨ Drugs can alter the course of the CVS illness, can change the signs and symptoms, can give rise to new CVS diseases and moreover some drugs have to be stopped before some procedures and investigations.

⇨ Patient has a h/o breathlessness and shows us that he is taking some diuretics and digoxin → think of CCF.

⇨ Patient has a h/o breathlessness and has a rotahaler in his pocket → think of asthma.

⇨ H/O acute chest pain responding to steroids → think of pericarditis.

⇨ H/O chest pain responding to some sublingual tablet (nitrate) → think of angina.

⇨ H/O sore throat, fever and severe bone pain responding to aspirin → think of acute rheumatic fever.

Drugs that can increase cardiovascular disease manifestations

(1) Myocardial infarction may be hampered if we concomitantly give nifedipine or hydralazine(↑myocardial work due to tachycardia), dipyridamole (↓coronary perfusion due to coronary steal phenomenon), ergot alkaloids(vasospasm), etc.

(2) Valvular heart diseases like MS or AS can be worsened if we give vasodilators to the patient as it causes tachycardia, decreased diastolic time, syncope and reduced BP.

(3) Congestive cardiac failure is worsened by calcium channel blockers (due to depression of myocardium), and drugs like steroids and NSAIDs (by causing ↑ salt and water retention).

It is important to note the intake of certain medications that can induce new cardiovascular symptoms like:

⇨ NSAIDs, hormonal therapy, cough drops, and ephedrine can cause new onset HYPERTENSION.

⇨ Excessive alcohol consumption, chemotherapeutic drugs(doxorubicin, bleomycin, cyclophosphamide), methyldopa, antibiotics(penicillin, sulfonamides tetracyclines), lithium, chloroquine can cause CARDIOMYOPATHY.

⇨ OC pills, phenformin can induce PAH.

⇨ Hydroxychloroquine, quinidine, antiarrhythmic drugs(amiodarone, procainamide, sotalol), erythromycin, ketoconazole can lead to QT PROLONGATION.

Side effects of some of the commonly used cardiovascular drugs

⇨ ACE inhibitors: Dry cough, hyperkalemia, raised creatinine(in renal artery stenosis)

⇨ Diuretics: Hypokalemia, dilutional hyponatremia, muscle cramps

⇨ Spironolactone: Hyperkalemia, gynecomastia, Erythema annulare centrifugum

⇨ Amiodarone: Lung fibrosis, liver dysfunction, thyroid disorders

⇨ Beta blockers: Bronchoconstriction, aggravation of diabetes mellitus, loss of libido, sleep disturbances

⇨ Heparin: Abnormal bleeding, osteoporosis

⇨ Aspirin: Dyspepsia, gut mucosal bleed

⇨ Digoxin: Vision abnormalities, gynecomastia, GI symptoms

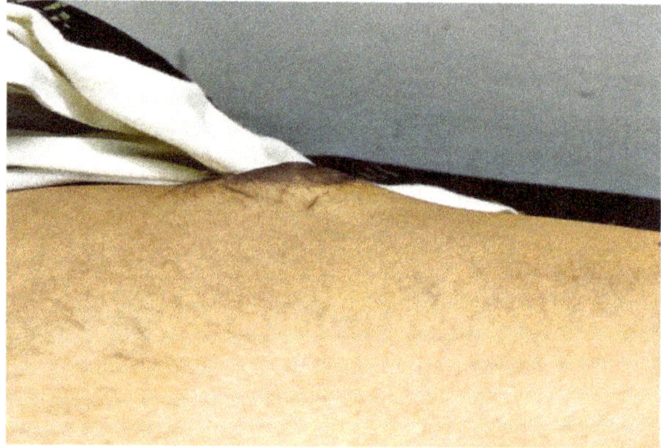

Fig. 1.5: Gynecomastia.

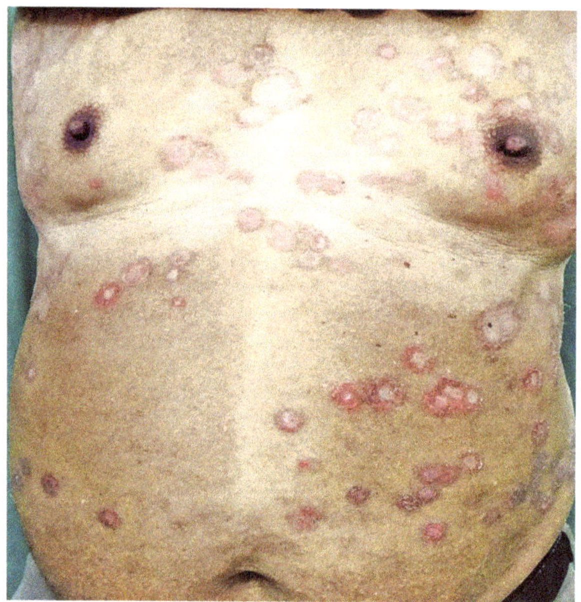

Fig. 1.6: Erythema annulare centrifugum (Courtesy: Dr. Som Lakhani, MD Skin and VD).

Family history and addiction history

- Family history is important for CAD and cardiomyopathies.
- H/O alcoholism is important for CAD, atrial fibrillation, dilated cardiomyopathy.
- H/O smoking is important for CAD.
- Valvular heart disease is evaluated with history of fever, prior sore throat, migratory polyarthritis, edema of the feet, palpitations, breathlessness, H/O taking white colored injections every 21 days(penicillin injections).
- Last but not the least, coronary risk factors should always be sought while taking the history like h/o diabetes, hypertension, obesity, hyperlipidemia, etc.

PALPITATION

It is an abnormal awareness of one's own heart beats.

Causes

Cardiovascular:

⇨ Regurgitant valve disorders like MR, AR, TR (due to ↑SV)

⇨ Congenital heart diseases like VSD, PDA, ARVD, TAPVC, Ebstein's anomaly.

⇨ Arrhythmic disorders like VT, SVT, atrial fibrillation (AF), sick sinus syndrome, malfunctioning pacemaker, hypertrophic cardiomyopathy, MVP.

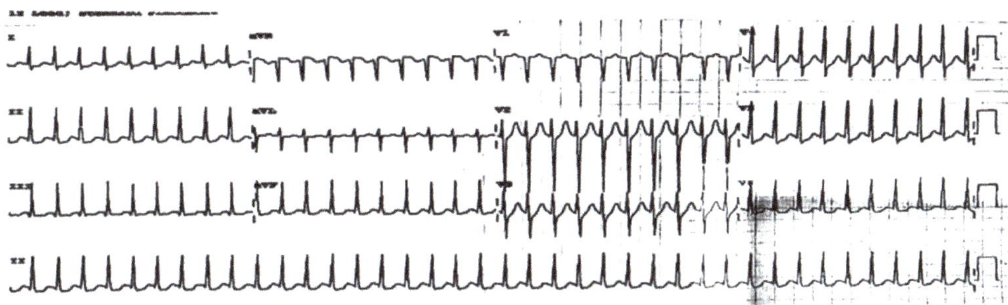

Fig. 1.7: Supraventricular tachycardia.

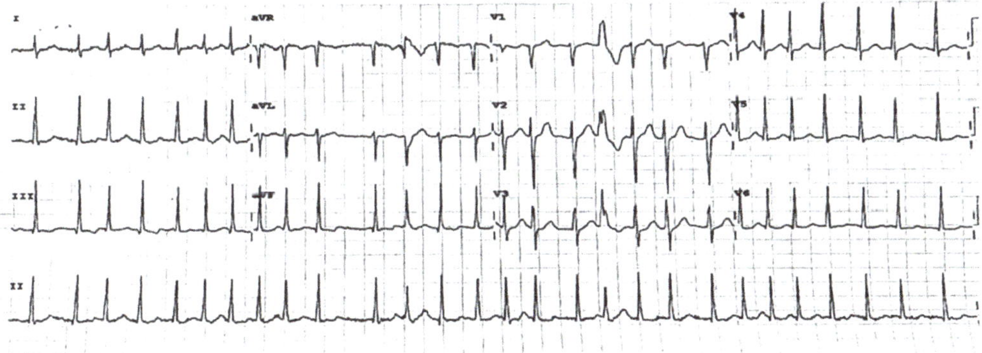

Fig. 1.8: Atrial fibrillation.

Non-cardiovascular:

⇨ Hyperdynamic states: Fever, hyperthyroidism, anemia, AV fistula, Paget's disease.

⇨ Drugs: Digoxin, tricyclic antidepressants, amphetamine, nitrates, nifedipine.

⇨ Metabolic: Hypoglycemia.

⇨ Psychogenic: Anxiety neurosis, panic attacks, depression.

Sustained palpitations

⇨ Indicates a state of volume overload

⇨ Seen in AR, MR, PDA, VSD, TAPVC, AF, anemia, AV fistula, psychosis.

Episodic palpitations

⇨ Arrhythmic disorders

⇨ Psychosis

⇨ Pheochromocytoma

⇨ Thyrotoxicosis, reduced sugar levels, drugs.

Sudden onet, sudden ending palpitations

⇨ AF

⇨ Paroxysmal atrial tachycardia

⇨ Atrial flutter

Gradual palpitations

⇨ Anxiety disorders

⇨ Sinus tachycardia

Palpitations precipitated by exercise

⇨ Shunts - VSD, ASD, PDA

⇨ Regurgitant lesions - AR, MR

⇨ Supraventricular rhythms, AF

Some causes of palpitations and their clinical clues

(1) **Regurgitant lesions like AR, TR** ⇨ Palpitations with neck throbbing.

(2) **Myocardial infarction, Pheochromocytoma, reduced sugar levels** ⇨ Palpitations with excessive perspiration.

(3) **Occasional pounding of the chest and inability to cope up with the breath** ⇨ Premature ventricular contractions.

(4) **Thyrotoxicosis** ⇨ Palpitations with loose stools.

(5) **PE, CCF** ⇨ Palpitations with breathlessness.

(6) **Sick sinus syndrome, reduced sugar levels** ⇨ Palpitations with syncope.

(7) **AF** ⇨ Nocturnal palpitations.

(8) **AV node tachycardia, pericarditis** ⇨ Positional palpitations.

(9) **SVT** ⇨ Childhood palpitations, and palpitations ending with vagal stimulation.

(10) **Catecholamine related palpitations** ⇨ Palpitations induced by stressful events.

SYNCOPE

⇨ Sudden unconsciousness lasting for a short interval of time and is related to acute cerebral hypoperfusion.

⇨ Manifested by facial pallor, perspiration, palpitations, vomiting, etc.

⇨ May suggest some serious disorders within the body.

Etiology

(1) Cerebral hypoperfusion
- Carotid sinus hypersensitivity (common in middle aged and elderly and leads to syncope on bending forward or head turning or wearing a shirt with tightly fit collar, etc)
- Vasovagal syncope
- Orthostatic hypotension (syncope on rising from the bed in the morning)
- Hypovolemic shock
- Drugs causing ↓BP like nitrates, antihypertensive drugs, etc.
- Traumatic brain injury, cerebrovascular accidents, epilepsy, etc.

(2) Cardiovascular causes (↓CO)
- Ventricular outflow obstruction: HOCM, AS, PS, PAH (all these causes syncope during exertion).
- Ventricular dysfunction: Myocardial infarction
- Filling defects of the ventricles: LA Myxomas (postural syncope), PE, syncope due to cough in smokers and obese, syncope during micturition.
- Abnormal heart rhythms: 3^0 heart blocks, AF, sick sinus syndrome.
- Excessive vagal stimulation reflexly during procedures like upper gastroscopy, bronchoscopy, peritoneal irritation, etc.

(3) Anoxia, ↓sugar level(may be associated with insulin use), hyperventilation.

(4) Hysteria: Common in females.

GENERAL EXAMINATION IN CARDIOLOGY

- General examination of every system should include a head to toe inspection or examination to see all the positive findings with respect to that particular system (CVS, CNS, PA or RS).
- One important thing that we usually miss in the initial part of the general examination of CVS is the **Waist circumference** and **Basal metabolic Index (BMI)**.
- **Waist circumference** is measured **at the level of the iliac crest in a horizontal plane** with a measuring tape.
- **BMI** is body mass (in kilograms) divided by the square of the body height (in meters), and is expressed in units of **kg/m^2**.
- **Normal BMI** ranges between **18.5 to 24.9**. A BMI under 18.5 suggests underweight status, 25 to 30 suggests overweight, 30 to 39.9 suggests obesity, and > 40 suggests morbid obesity.
- Central(abdominal) obesity is more commonly associated with CAD compared to generalized obesity.
- Obesity can be associated with a number of syndromes which leads to increased cardiovascular complications. Some of them are:
  - → **Pickwickian syndrome:** obesity, hypoventilation, secondary polycythemia, somnolence, cyanosis, **pulmonary hypertension, and ↑ PVR**.
  - → **Metabolic syndrome**: obesity (waist circumference > 102 cm for men and > 88 cm for women), high triglyceride level (> or = to 150 mg%), decreased HDL (< 40 mg% in men and < 50 mg% in women), ↑ blood pressure (> 130/85 mmHg), ↑ fasting blood sugar (> or = to 100 mg%).
  - → **Cushing's syndrome**: obesity, buffalo hump, moon facies, purple striae on abdomen, hirsutism, osteoporosis, diabetes mellitus, acne.
  - → **Laurence-Moon-Biedl syndrome**: obesity, retinitis pigmentosa, polydactyly (multiple digits), mental retardation, hypogonadism and **congenital heart diseases**.
  - → **Hypothyroidism**
  - → **Frohlich's syndrome**: "girdle" type obesity, narrow fingers, absent axillary and pubic hairs, effeminate voice, and hypotonia.
  - → **Hand-Schuller-Christian disease:** obesity, exophthalmos, dwarfism, hypoplasia of gonads, **diabetes mellitus**.
- A BMI between 25 and 34.9 kg/m^2, Waist circumference > 102 cm (men) and > 88 cm (women) is associated with ↑ risk of coronary artery diseases (CAD), hypertension, diabetes mellitus, and hyperlipidemia.
- A body weight below normal (**underweight** or BMI < 18.5) may be **associated with chronic heart failure** (cardiac cachexia), diabetes mellitus, thyrotoxicosis, etc.

- Underweight status can be diagnosed with the help of skin fold thickness by skin calipers.
- **Baldness** (male pattern) can also be linked to increased likelihood of coronary artery disease **(CAD)**. [Medical news today - "Baldness linked to higher risk of coronary heart disease"......Sarah Glynn on April 4, 2013.]
- However, only vertex or crown head baldness is associated with high risk of CAD.
- **Hamilton Scale** is used to **grade the severity of baldness** and as the severity increases, the risk of CAD increases as well.
- Risk of CAD is increased by:
  → 48% in severe vertex baldness
  → 36% in moderate vertex baldness
  → 18% in mild vertex baldness
- It is thought that baldness increases the risk of CAD through:
  → Chronic inflammation
  → Increased testosterone sensitivity
  → Resistance to insulin.

GENERAL BUILT-STATURE

Built and stature includes:

→ Height, Lower and Upper segments

→ Arm span

→ Body mass index (BMI) (Discussed above already)

→ Waist circumference (Discussed above already)

Height

- **Upper segment:** From top of the head to upper border of the symphysis pubis (pubic ramus).
- **Lower segment:** From top of the pubic symphysis to soles.
- Upper segment/Lower segment ratio is equal after the age of 10 years.
- **Arm span**: Distance between the tips of the middle fingers of both the hands when the arms are stretched horizontally out from the body.
- **Stature = Upper segment + Lower segment**
- **Arm span/ Height ratio ≑ 1.05**

  Checking the height is important to check whether the patient has a tall stature or short stature, because both the conditions may be associated with various CVS abnormalities.

Tall stature

Height > 2 standard deviations of the mean for the age and race.

D/D of tall stature

→ Constitutional and pituitary giants: tall stature with upper segment equal to lower segment.

→ Marfan syndrome, Homocystinuria, Eunuchoidism, Klinefelter's syndrome: tall stature with lower segment > upper segment and arm span > height.

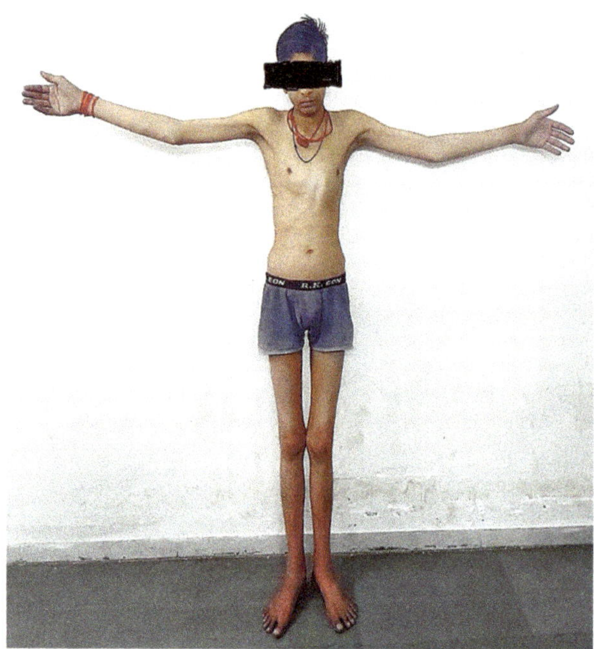

Fig. 1.9: A patient of Marfan's syndrome with tall stature and increased arm span.

Gigantism

- Generalized, symmetrical overgrowth with ↑ skeletal length and the height far in excess of the normal.
- **In india**, we suspect gigantism if the height is in excess of **6 feet**. (Worldwide it is 6.6 feet)

Constitutional gigantism

Perfectly proportional body with normal mental, physical, and sexual functions.

Hyper Pituitary gigantism: Excessive anterior pituitary functioning before fusion of the epiphyses. Body is well proportioned with normal sexual function, splanchnomegaly, raised intracranial tension, polyuria and glycosuria.

Marfan syndrome

Disorder of connective tissue. AD in inheritance. Incidence of 2–3 per 10, 000. There is an abnormality of fibrillin, a supporting scaffold for elastin in the body. Fibrillin- found in other tissues also like the lung, dura, skin, tendons, ciliary zonules of the lens, myocardium, heart valves and periosteum.Cases should be regularly assessed by echocardiography, optometry and skeletal survey. A proper family history and screening of family members can also give clues to the disease.

Ghent criteria for diagnosing Marfan's syndrome

Major criteria required in 2 organ systems and minor criterion in a 3rd system

System involved	Major criteria	Minor criteria
Family history	Independent in parent or child or sibling	None
CVS	Dilatation of aortic root, Dissection of Asc. aorta	MVP, mitral valve calcification (< 40 years), pulm.artery dilatation, Desc. aorta dissection
Genetics	FBN1 mutation	None
Pulmonary		Spontaneous pneumothorax, apex bulla
Ocular	Upward dislocation of the lens (ectopia lentis)	2 of the following: flat cornea, elongated globe myopia, hypoplasia of the iris or ciliary muscle
Skeletal	Minimum 4 to be present out of the following: Pectus excavatum necessitating surgery, pectus carinatum, flat foot, positive Walker-Murdock (wrist) sign or Steinberg (thumb) sign, scoliosis > 20° or spondylolisthesis, arm span/height ratio > 1.05, protrusio acetabuli by radiography, ↓ extension elbows (< 170°)	2 to 3 major, or 1 major and 2 minor signs should be present: pectus excavatum (moderate), high arched palate, typical facial features, hypermobility of joints
Skin		Stretch marks (shoulder), recurrent or incisional hernia
CNS	Lumbosacral dural ectasia by CT or MRI	

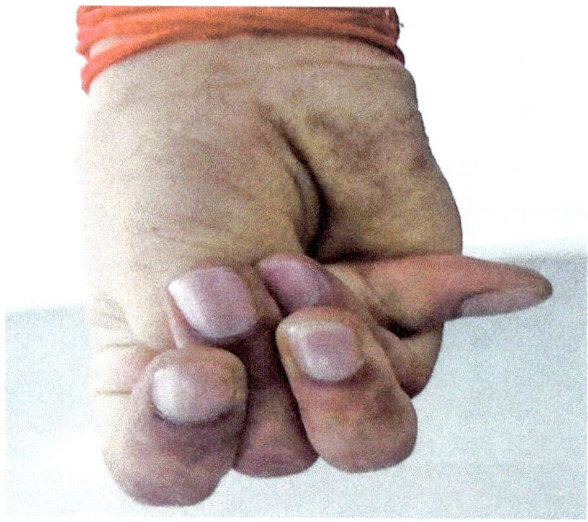

Fig. 1.10: Thumb sign in Marfan's syndrome.

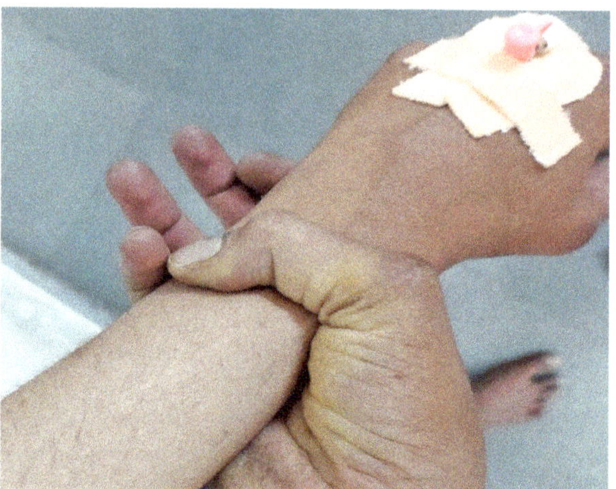

Fig. 1.11: Wrist sign in Marfan's syndrome.

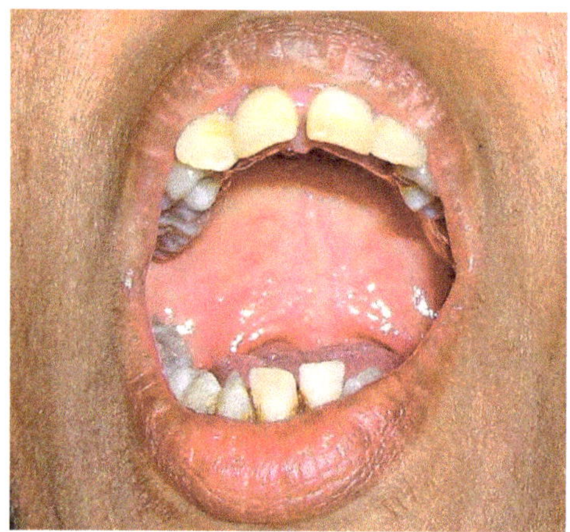

Fig. 1.12: High arched palate (Courtesy: Dr. Rajesh U Patel, Sai Drashti Eye Hospital, Bharuch).

CVS diseases associated with Marfan syndrome are

- → Dilatation of aortic root with subsequent dissection of the ascending aorta
- → Dilatation of the main pulmonary artery; diagnostic especially when the patient is < 40 year old
- → MR/ MVP/ Mitral annular calcification
- → Dilatation of descending aorta and subsequent dissection
- → Prolapse of the tricuspid valve
- → LV dysfunction
- → WPW syndrome and atrial fibrillation
- → Aneurysms of the coronary arteries
- → ASD

It should be very clear from the above description that whenever we examine a case of Marfan syndrome, we should always check (from cardiology point of view):

→ Weight and Height

→ BP

→ CVS auscultation to check for any murmur(s)

→ ECG

→ 2D Echo every 6 to 12 months to see for LV dilatation, pulmonary artery, aortic root, etc.

Homocystinuria: Inborn error of amino acid metabolism where homocysteine accumulates in the blood and produces a slowly evolving clinical syndrome.

Homocystinuria type-1

→ deficiency of cystathionine ß synthase.

→ delayed milestones, ectopia lentis, mental retardation (progressive), skeletal abnormalities like Marfan syndrome and thromboembolism.

Homocystinuria type-II

→ defect in methylcobalamin formation

→ triad of megaloblastic anemia, homocystinuria and hypermethioninemia

Homocystinuria type-III

→ lack of methyltetrahydrofolate reductase

→ homocysteinemia, homocystinuria and low to low normal methionine levels.

CVS diseases associated with Homocystinurla are

→ Ischaemic heart disease

→ Cerebrovascular disease

→ Pulmonary embolism

Klinefelter's syndrome: (XXX/XXY). Eunuchoid appearance, tall height, testes-small, azoospermia, mental retardation, gynecomastia.

CVS diseases associated with Klinefelter's syndrome are

→ LV diastolic dysfunction

→ Thrombosis and leg ulcers

→ Chronotropic incompetence and decreased maximal oxygen consumption

→ Congenital anomalies - ASD, VSD, MVP, Acute MR, PAPVC with PAH, Hypertrophic cardiomyopathy.

SHARP'S SYNDROME ⇒ Klinefelter's syndrome + Mixed connective tissue disease

Short stature

Height < 2 standard deviations of the mean for the age and race.

For India, height < 4 feet is considered short stature.

D/D of short stature

→ Hereditary or Constitutional dwarfism

→ Endocrine dwarfism: Cretin, Pituitary dwarf, Frohlich's syndrome, Cushing's syndrome

→ Genetic causes: Turner's syndrome, Noonan syndrome, Hurler's syndrome, Morquios syndrome, etc.

Hereditary/Constitutional dwarfism: For example Gurkhas, African pygmies, Lapps, etc. Except for the short height, the hereditary dwarf is normal in all other aspects. They have normal levels of Growth hormone and Gonadotropin.

Endocrine dwarfism

→ **Cretinism:** Due to hypothyroidism. They have short stature, mental retardation, large size head, coarse hair, dry skin, large tongue, puffy eyes, thickened lips, spade-like hands, infantile genitals, pot belly. The ratio of upper segment/lower segment is < 1.

→ **Frohlich's syndrome:** Also called Dystrophia **adiposogenitalis**. Occurs due to pituitary or hypothalamic dysfunction. The patient has normal intelligence, underdeveloped genitals, short stature, and obesity.

→ **Pituitary dwarfism:** Although the child is normal at birth but later shows a slower rate of growth and develops short limbs, decreased axillary and pubic hairs, underdeveloped genitals, normal intelligence and shows infantilism.

→ **Cushing's syndrome:** Buffalo hump, obesity, moon like face, hirsutism, purple striae on the abdomen, hypertension, and impaired glucose tolerance.

Genetic dwarfism

Turner syndrome (45X): Short stature female, webbing of the neck, shield chest with widely spaced nipples, low set hair line, sexual infantilism, normal intelligence, premature ovarian failure.

CVS diseases associated with Turner syndrome are

→ Bicuspid aortic valve (15% to 30%)

→ Aortic coarctation(post ductal type) (7% to 18%)

→ PAPVC

→ Left Superior vena cava

→ Elongated transverse aorta

→ Dilated head and neck arteries

Noonan syndrome

Autosomal dominant. Normal chromosomes. Facial abnormalities, congenital heart diseases, short stature, webbed neck, chest deformities, undescended testes, ptosis, mental impairment.

CVS diseases associated with Noonan syndrome are

→ Pulmonary stenosis with/without dysplastic pulmonary valve

→ Hypertrophic cardiomyopathy

→ ASD

→ AV septal defects

→ Left-sided obstructive lesions

→ TOF

→ PDA

Ellis-van Creveld syndrome

Chondral and ectodermal dysplasia. Short ribs, shortening of long bones, dysplastic nails and teeth, lip tie, polydactyly, growth retardation, and ectodermal and heart defects. Cognitive and motor development is normal.

CVS diseases associated with Ellis-van Creveld syndrome are

→ Common atrium

→ ASD

→ Persistent Left Superior vena cava

→ Abnormal pulmonary venous connection

Short limb dwarfism ⇒ Achondroplasia, Osteogenesis imperfecta, Diastrophic dwarfism, Hypochondroplasia, Pseudoachondroplasia.

Short trunk dwarfism ⇒ Spondylocostal dysostosis, Spondyloepiphyseal dysplasia tarda, Kniest dysplasia Spondyloepiphyseal dysplasia congenita.

Posture and Gesture of the patient

Posture of the patient and the gesture he/she makes while telling the history to you can give real clues to the diagnosis.

→ A patient who sits quietly after walking some distance can be seen in Angina pectoris.

→ A restless patient with excessive sweating can indicate Myocardial infarction.

→ Patient who is comfortable in the upright posture and becomes breathless in a lying down position can occur in Left heart failure (also in ascites, asthma, pregnancy etc).

→ Patient who is comfortable in a seated and bending forward position(prayer posture) can indicate Pericarditis.

→ Patient holding a clenched fist in front of the sternum is called as "Levine's sign" and indicates ischemic cardiac pain.

→ If the patient can pinpoint his chest by a single finger and around the mammary region then there is a high likelihood that the chest pain is of Non cardiac origin.

→ A patient who climbs upon himself while getting up from the sitting position is called "Gower's sign", commonly seen in Duchen's muscular dystrophy which can be associated with Cardiomyopathies.

THE HEAD AND NECK IN GENERAL EXAMINATION OF THE CVS

FACE

Many times, the facial look of the patient can give you a hint about the probable diagnosis of the CVS disease.

Facial dysmorphism are the facial abnormalities that occur due to abnormalities of the ears (low set/high set), teeth, hair line (low/high), lips (thick/thin), nose (broad/flat etc), neck (webbed/short), interpupillary distance (hypertelorism/hypotelorism), epicanthal folds, etc.

Here I mention some of the diseases that are associated with facial dysmorphism and cardiovascular abnormalities: -

Trisomy 21 (Downs syndrome) (Mongoloid Face): Flat face with flat and broad bridge of nose, almond shaped eyes with upward slant (inner epicanthal folds), short neck, small ears, large tongue, small hands, single palmar crease, incurved little finger, tiny white spots on the iris (Brushfields spots), strabismus, hypotonia, short height, mental retardation.

CVS diseases associated with Down's syndrome are

→ Endocardial cushion defects

→ VSD

→ ASD

→ TOF

Turner and Noonan syndrome: Hypertelorism, downslanting palpebral fissures, drooping of the eyelids, low-set posteriorly rotated ears, webbed neck, mild developmental delay, cryptorchidism in males (Noonan syndrome), abnormalities of the thorax, feeding difficulties in infancy, abnormal bleeding, and lymphatic dysplasia.

CVS abnormalities of Turner and Noonan syndromes have already been described earlier.

Cri du chat syndrome: Round asymmetrical face, strabismus, hypertelorism, small philtrum, inferiorly turned corners of the mouth, small jaws, low set ears, epicanthal folds, down slant of palpebral fissures, etc.

CVS diseases associated with Cri du chat syndrome are

→ ASD

→ VSD

→ PDA

William syndrome(Elfin facies): Epicanthal folds, depressed and broad nose, periorbital edema, anteverted nares, short palpebral fissure, prominent lips, long philtrum, hoarse voice, ears that are low set, ↑interpupillary distance, hypercalcemia.

CVS diseases associated with William syndrome are

→ Supravalvular aortic stenosis

→ Peripheral pulmonary stenosis

Acromegaly (Ape like face): Pronounced mandibular prognathism, thick broad nose, thick lips, prominence of supraorbital ridges, prominent facial lines, macroglossia, hypertrichosis, large hands and feet.

CVS diseases associated with Acromegaly are:

→ Concentric hypertrophy (MC)

→ Disorders of cardiac rhythm

→ Cardiomyopathies

→ Hypertension

Kabuki syndrome: Microcephaly, cleft palate, hypotonia, nystagmus, strabismus, short stature, scoliosis, short fifth finger, high arched palate, poor dentition.

CVS diseases associated with Kabuki syndrome are

→ ASD

→ CoA

→ AS

→ Hypoplastic left heart syndrome

→ MS

DiGeorge syndrome: Cleft palate, bifid uvula, asymmetric crying facies, hypertelorism, microcephaly, low-set ears, wide-set eyes, underdeveloped chin, narrow palpebral fissures, hypocalcemia, renal anomalies, feeding and swallowing problems, hearing loss, seizures, skeletal anomalies, and immune deficiencies.

CVS diseases associated with DiGeorge syndrome are

→ TOF

→ PDA

→ Interrupted aortic arch

→ Truncus arteriosus

→ VSD

Alagille syndrome: Prominent forehead, long nose, deep eyes, prominent chin, low set ears.

CVS diseases associated with Alagille syndrome are

→ Peripheral pulmonary stenosis

→ Pulmonary stenosis

→ TOF

Mucopolysaccharidosis type 1 (Hurler's syndrome): Gargoyle-like faces. Broad nasal bridge, full cheeks, thick lips, enlarged tongue, coarse hair, hirsutism, macrocephaly, corneal opacities, hypertelorism, small misaligned teeth.

CVS diseases associated with Hurler's syndrome are

→ Coronary artery disease

→ AR

→ MR

Cushing's syndrome (Moon like face): Buffalo hump, obesity, moon like face, hirsutism, purple striae on the abdomen, hypertension, and impaired glucose tolerance.

CVS diseases associated with Cushing's syndrome are

→ Metabolic syndrome

→ Atherosclerosis

→ Coronary artery disease

→ Heart failure

→ Cerebrovascular accident

Fetal alcohol syndrome

Hypoplasia of the maxilla, small nose, microcephaly, short palpebral fissure, thin upper lip.

CVS diseases associated with Fetal alcohol syndrome are

→ ASD

→ VSD

→ TOF

→ PDA

Congenital Rubella: Microcephaly, microphthalmia, premature cataract.

CVS diseases associated with Congenital Rubella are

→ Pulmonary artery stenosis

→ PDA

Hypothyroidism: Swollen face, dry skin, hoarseness of voice, large tongue, madarosis, increased weight, menorrhagia, constipation, cold intolerance.

CVS diseases associated with Hypothyroidism are

→ Diastolic hypertension

→ Pericardial effusion

→ Atherosclerosis

Hyperthyroidism: Staring look, all eyes signs(discussed later), unexplained weight loss despite normal appetite, heat intolerance, moist skin.

CVS diseases associated with Hyperthyroidism are

→ Tachycardia

→ Atrial fibrillation

→ High cardiac output state

→ Wide pulse pressure

→ Means-Lerman scratch

Werner's syndrome: Leads to premature aging of subcutaneous tissues, loss of hair, graying of hair, cataract, ulcers on the legs.

CVS diseases associated with Werner's syndrome are:

→ Atherosclerosis

Apart from facial dysmorphism (described above), we should always keep an eye on the other facial findings that would help us arrive at a diagnosis with a cardiovascular perspective.

Swelling of the face

→ Swelling of the face on bending forward points at a diagnosis of constrictive pericarditis.

→ Swelling of the face with engorgement of the chest veins indicates SVC obstruction syndrome (commonly due to bronchogenic carcinoma).

→ Hypothyroidism is a common cause of facial swelling.

Malar flush on the cheeks is a purple-red discoloration commonly seen in Mitral stenosis and is due to CO_2 retention and its vasodilatory effects. It can also be seen in SLE and Polycythemia rubra vera.

Periorbital swelling may be seen in patients of renal failure which may be associated with hypertension very frequently.

Butterfly rash on the face is seen in SLE which can be associated with a number of CVS diseases like premature atherosclerosis, myocarditis, pericarditis, Libman-Sacks endocarditis, heart blocks (in babies of SLE affected mothers), etc.

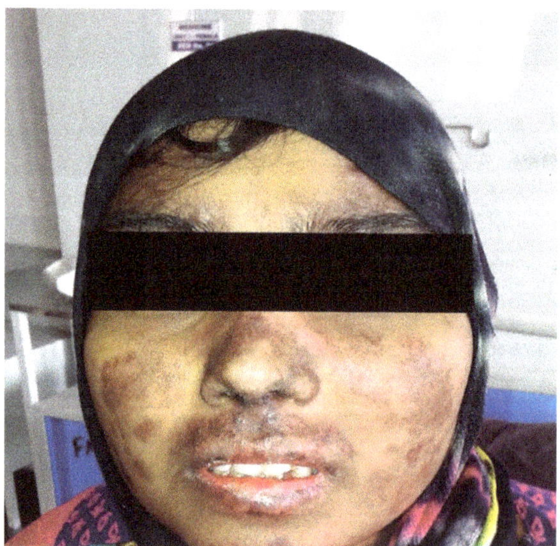

Fig. 1.13: Butterfly rash in SLE.

EYES

Examination of the eyes should start with the general appearance like sunken or protruded and then should proceed for higher things like normal or excessive distance between the eyes, then looking for the conjunctiva, eyelids, sclera, cornea, retina etc.

Sunken eyes or Enophthalmos can occur in patients who have hypovolemic shock due to diarrhea or can also be seen in cardiac cachexia.

Protruding eyes or Exophthalmos is more commonly seen in Hyperthyroidism. However, a pulsatile exophthalmos is seen in severe tricuspid regurgitation.

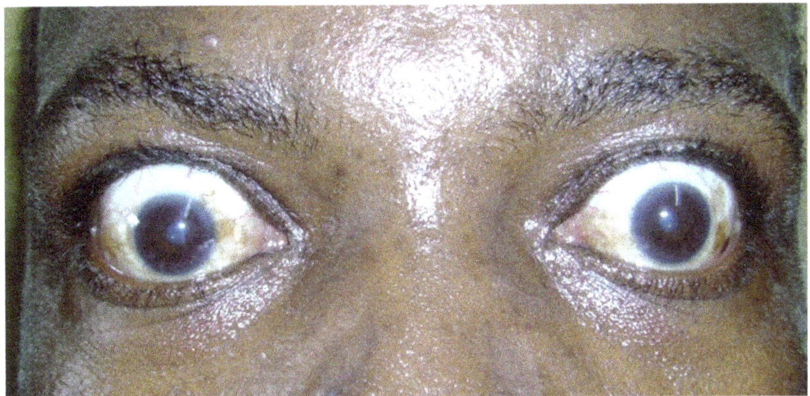

Fig. 1.14: Exophthalmos (Courtesy: Dr. Rajesh U Patel, Sai Drashti Eye Hospital, Bharuch).

Hypertelorism (↑Interpupillary distance) is seen in diseases like Turner's syndrome, Noonan syndrome, Hurler syndrome, William syndrome (all described earlier), LEOPARD syndrome, and Klippel-Feil syndrome.

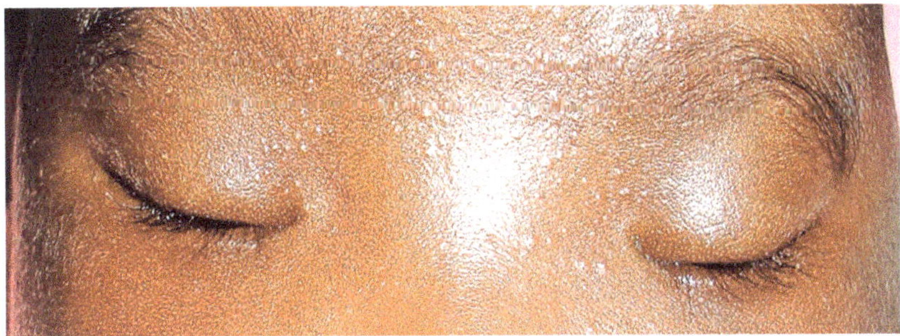

Fig. 1.15: Hypertelorism (Courtesy: Dr. Rajesh U Patel, Sai Drashti Eye Hospital, Bharuch).

LEOPARD syndrome ⇒ ***L****entigines* (multiple), ***E****CG* conduction abnormalities, ***O****cular* hypertelorism, ***P****ulmonic* stenosis, ***A****bnormal* genitals, ***R****etarded* growth, and ***D****eafness* (sensorineural).

CVS diseases associated with LEOPARD syndrome are

→ Electrocardiographic anomalies and progressive conduction anomalies (Currently the most common)

→ Pulmonary valve stenosis (Most common according to previous reports)

→ Hypertrophic cardiomyopathy

Klippel-Feil syndrome ⇒ Short neck, low posterior hairline, fused cervical vertebrae, restricted neck movements, cleft palate, strabismus, deafness.

CVS disease associated with Klippel-Feil syndrome are

→ VSD

Eyelids examination helps us clinically detect some CVS diseases like:

→ Drooping of the upper eyelids (**Ptosis**): Ptosis (external ophthalmoplegia) in association with pigmentary retinopathy and cardiac conduction disorders (like complete heart block) is seen as a triad in Kearns-Sayre syndrome which is a mitochondrial myopathy with onset before the age of 20 years. Other clinical findings are ataxia, deafness and diabetes mellitus.

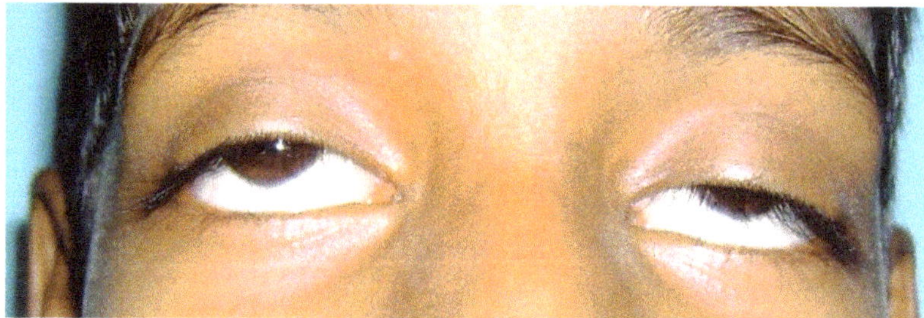

Fig. 1.16: Ptosis (Courtesy: Dr. Rajesh U Patel, Sai Drashti Eye Hospital, Bharuch).

→ **Lid lag** is a known finding of thyrotoxicosis which is associated with cardiovascular complications described previously.(**)

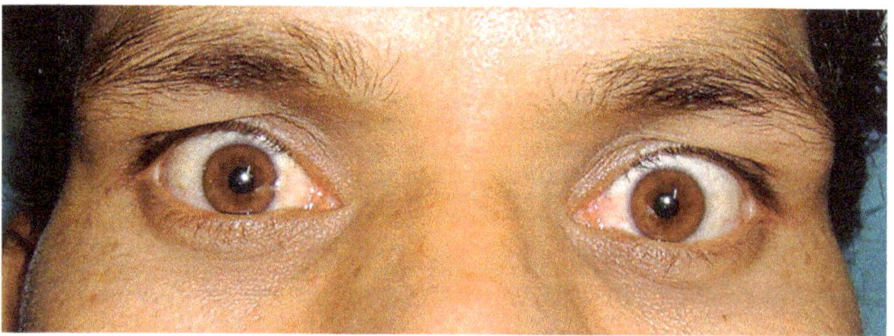

Fig. 1.17: Lid lag (Courtesy: Dr.Rajesh U Patel, Sai Drashti Eye Hospital, Bharuch).

→ Yellowish pink nodules seen near the inner canthus of eyes called as **Xanthelasma** may be an indicator of Dyslipidemia and coronary artery disease (not diagnostic).(@@)

(**) Other eye signs associated with Thyrotoxicosis are

- Dalrymple's sign: Retraction of the upper eyelid
- Enroth's sign: Swelling of eyelids
- Abadie's sign: Spastic elevator muscle of upper eyelid
- Ballet's sign: Extraocular muscle paralysis
- Becker's sign: Abnormal retinal arterial pulsations
- Boston's sign: Jerky movement of upper eyelid on downward gaze
- Gifford's sign: Difficult eversion of upper eyelid
- Cowen's sign: Consensual pupillary reflex hippus
- Griffith's sign: Lower lid lag on upper gaze
- Goldzeiher's sign: Conjunctival injection (temporal)
- Hertoghe's sign: Loss of eyebrows laterally
- Jellinek's sign: Hyperpigmented superior eyelid fold
- von Graefe's sign: Upper lid lag on lower gaze
- Joffroy's sign: Absent forehead creases on upward gaze
- Jendrassik's sign: Limited abduction and rotation of the eyeball
- Knies's sign: Uneven dilation of pupils in dim light
- Loewi's sign: Quick dilatation of pupils after instillation of 1: 1000 adrenaline
- Kocher's sign: Spasm and retraction of upper eyelid on fixation
- Mann's sign: Eyes seem to be situated at different levels because of tanned skin
- Mean sign: ↑ scleral show on upward gaze
- Payne–Trousseau's sign: Globe dislocation
- Mobius's sign: Loss of convergence
- Riesman's sign: Bruit over the eyelids
- Pochin's sign: ↓ amplitude of blinking
- Rosenbach's sign: Thin tremors when eyelids are closed
- Stellwag's sign: Incomplete blinking
- Suker's sign: Difficulty to maintain fixation on extreme lateral gaze
- Wilder's sign: Abduction to adduction movement produces jerking of the eyes

(@@) Clinical signs of Dyslipidemia are

- Xanthelasma
- Corneal arcus
- Xanthoma
- Deep earlobe crease (Frank sign)
- Locomotor brachialis (Also a peripheral sign of AR)
- Hepatosplenomegaly

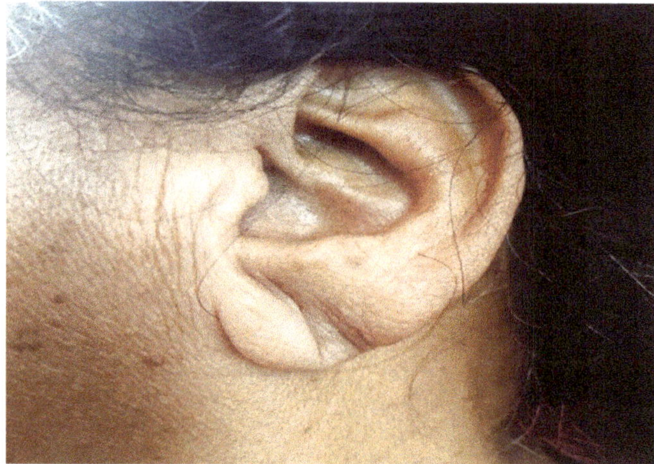

Fig. 1.18: Ear lobe crease or frank's sign.

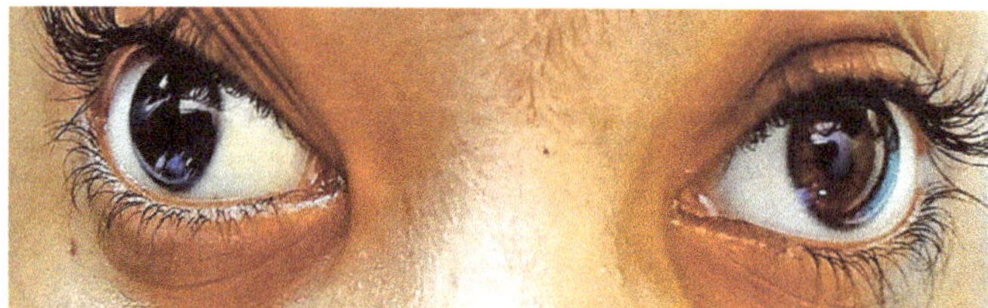

Fig. 1.19: Corneal arcus at lower aspect in Familial hypercholesterolemia (Courtesy: Dr. Sriranga R).

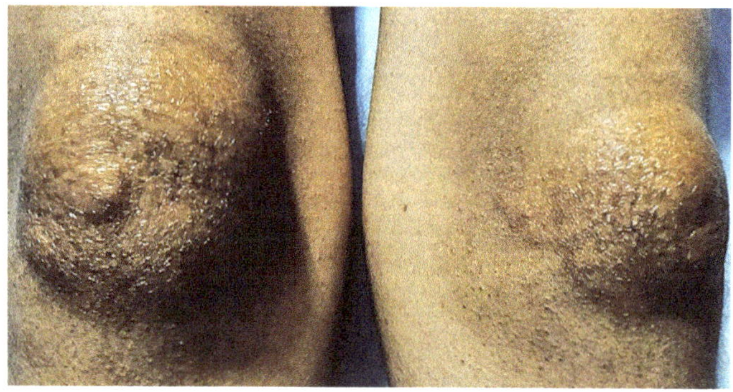

Fig. 1.20: Bilateral knee xanthomas in Familial hypercholesterolemia (Courtesy: Dr. Sriranga R).

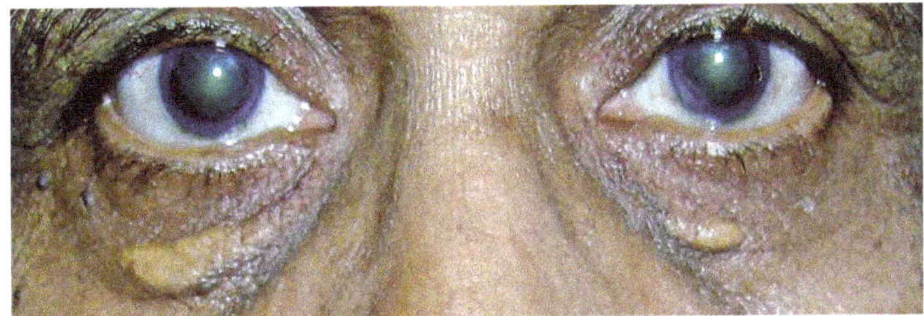

Fig. 1.21: Xanthelasma (Courtesy: Dr. Rajesh U Patel, Sai Drashti Eye Hospital, Bharuch).

Conjunctival examination in Cardiology

→ Pallor: High output failure in anemia.

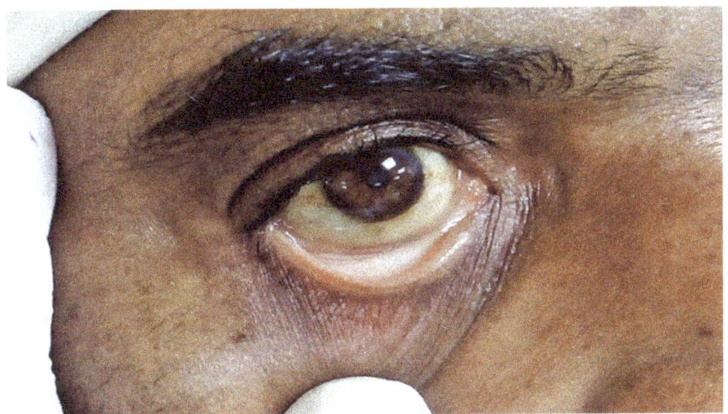

Fig. 1.22: Pallor seen in lower sclera.

Pallor seen in lower sclera

→ Conjunctivitis: Reiter's disease is associated with the triad of Conjunctivitis, Urethritis, and Arthritis. Cardiac lesions seen in Reiter's disease are Pericarditis, Myocarditis (rarely) and AV conduction defects (Most commonly First degree AV block)

→ Conjunctival petechiae may occur in Infective endocarditis and may resemble microemboli or vasculitis.

Sclera should be examined for:

→ Icterus: Jaundice in cardiology can be attributed to ischemic hepatopathy secondary to Heart failure or at times due to hemolysis from prosthetic heart valves.

→ Blue sclera: Noted in Osteogenesis imperfecta (MVP, AR, Aortic dissection), Marfan's syndrome (described above), Ehlers-Danlos syndrome (TOF, ASD, Regurgitant lesions).

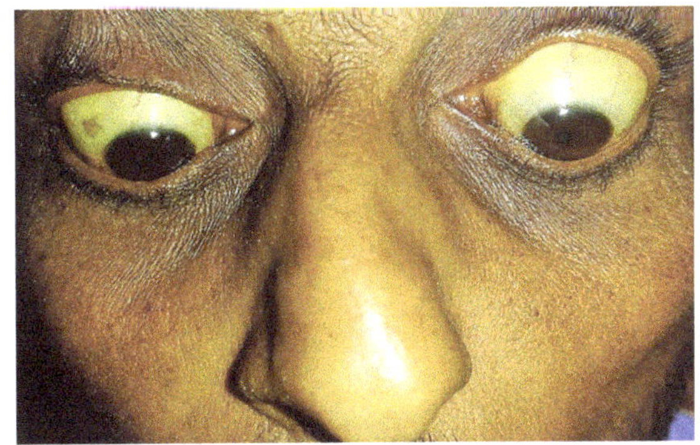

Fig. 1.23: Deep icterus with yellowing of the skin as well.

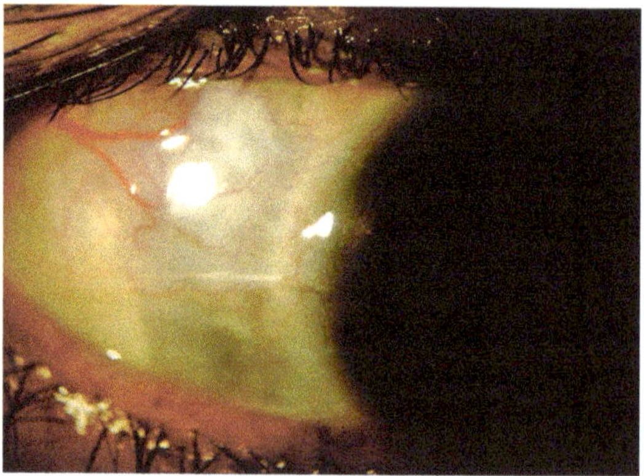

Fig. 1.24: Deep icterus with yellowing of the skin as well.

Corneal findings in cardiovascular diseases includes:

→ Corneal clouding: Mucopolysaccharidoses (MPS) I (Hurler: CAD, AR, MR)), IV (Morquio: MR, AR)), VI (Maroteaux-Lamy: Mitral and Aortic valve disease, PH), VII.

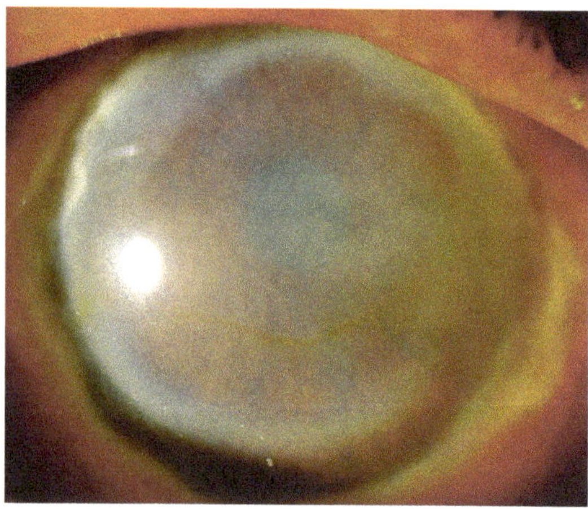

Fig. 1.25: Cloudy cornea (Courtesy: Dr. Rajesh U Patel, Sai Drashti Eye Hospital, Bharuch).

→ Corneal arcus: A known sign of hyperlipidemia in those < 50 years of age. Lipid deposits near the corneoscleral limbus but there is a small lipid-free zone from the limbus called the lucid interval of Vogt. Usually begins on the superior and inferior poles of the cornea and often progresses to form a complete ring without visual impairment.

→ Flat cornea: Marfan's syndrome

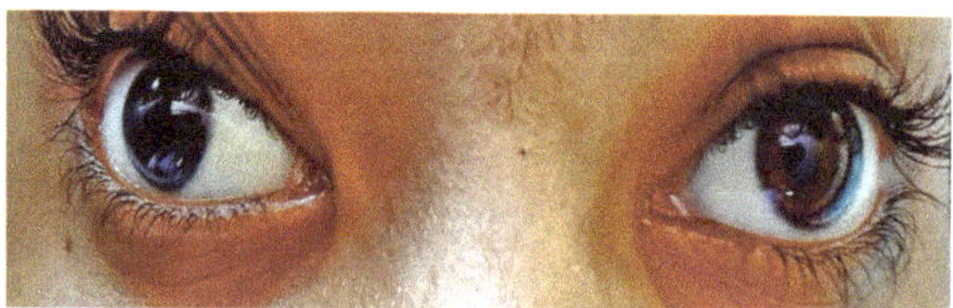

Fig. 1.26: Corneal arcus in Familial hypercholesterolemia (Courtesy: Dr. Sriranga R).

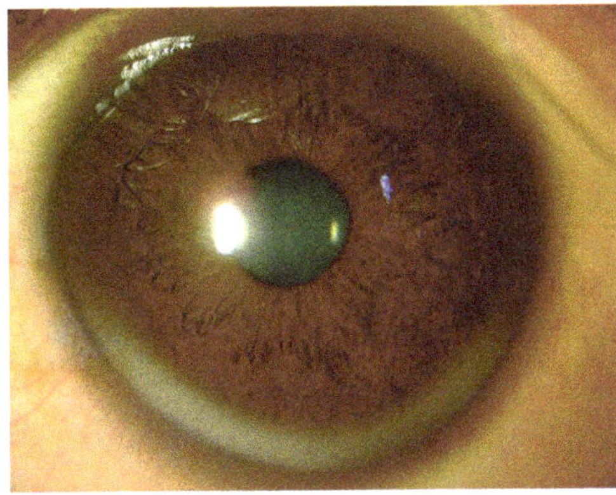

Fig. 1.27: Corneal arcus (Courtesy: Dr. Rajesh U Patel, Sai Drashti Eye Hospital, Bharuch).

Iris examination

→ Brushfields spots: (Indian Pediatrics 2002; 39: 97;BrushField spots)

White or yellow colored spots seen on the anterior surface of iris. Seen in about 85% of blue eyed patients of trisomy 21. Brushfield spots are less appreciable in Indians due to dark eyes. Brushfield spots should be differentiated from "Kunkmann Wolffian" bodies, which are less distinct, lesser in number and placed more peripherally than Brushfield spots without associated facial dysmorphism.

→ Coloboma:

Keyhole shaped defect in iris leading to an abnormal shape of the pupil. Coloboma of iris is seen in some syndromes that can be associated with heart diseases and defects.

- Mucopolysaccharidosis VII (Sly syndrome)
- CHARGE syndrome: Coloboma of iris or retina or choroid or disc, heart defects (conotruncal defects, AV canal defects, aortic arch anomalies), choanal atresia, retarded growth and development, genital abnormalities(labial hypoplasia, cryptorchidism, micropenis, hypogonadotrophic hypogonadism) and ear anomalies.

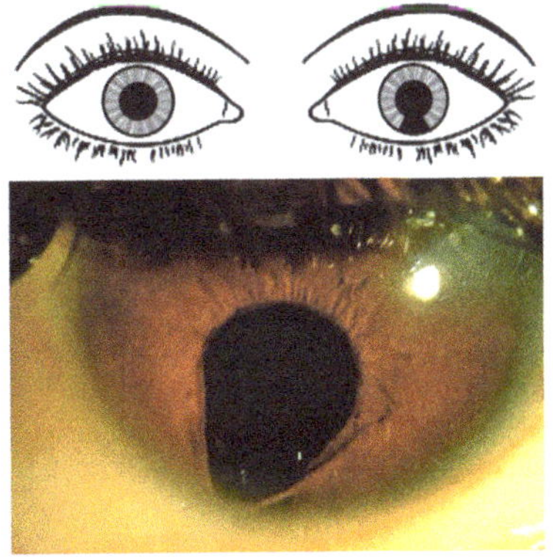

Fig. 1.28: Coloboma iris (Courtesy: Dr. Rajesh U Patel, Sai Drashti Eye Hospital, Bharuch).

- "Cat eye" syndrome: Coloboma of the iris and choroid (Cat eye appearance), anal atresia, abnormal genitourinary tract, ear anomalies, cardiac defects like TOF, TAPVC, Tricuspid atresia, ASD, VSD.

Pupils

Syphilis is one infection that can affect the pupils and has cardiovascular impact as well.

Argyll Robertson pupils are irregular and small pupils not reacting to light but have preserved accommodation reflexes.

It reflects involvement of the base of the brain.

Cardiovascular involvements in Syphilis include Aortitis, Aortic regurgitation, and Aortic aneurysms (Ascending aorta and arch), and stenosis of coronary ostium.

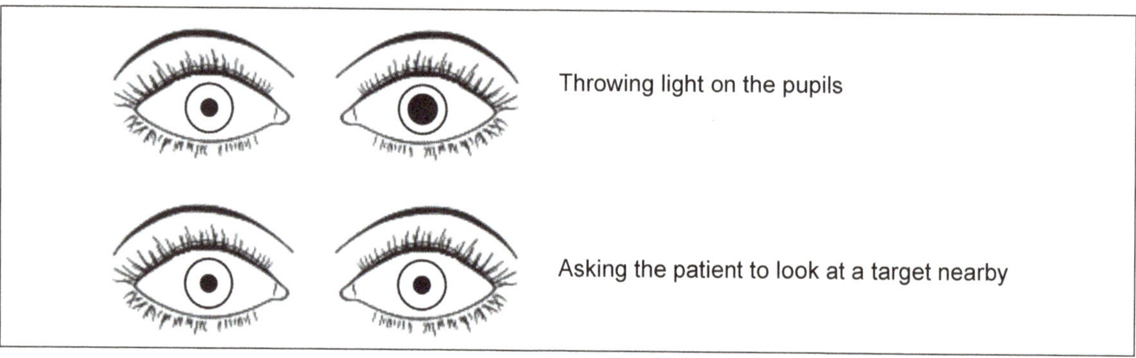

Fig. 1.29: Argyll Robertson pupil.

Lens

Young patients with Cataract are at increased risk of developing IHD.

Congenital Rubella, Werner's syndrome: Premature cataract (described earlier).

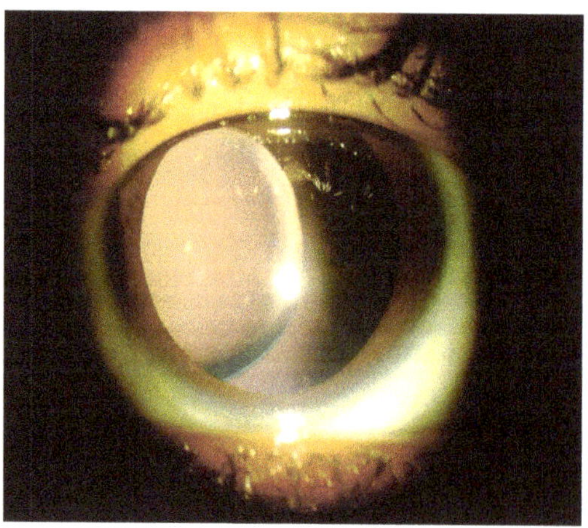

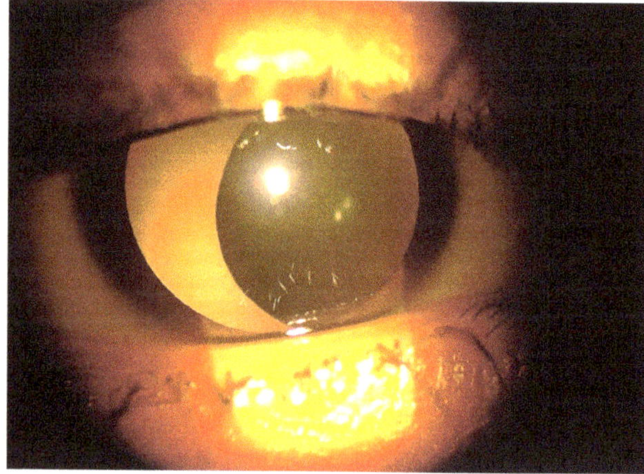

Fig. 1.30: Ectopia lentis (Courtesy: Dr.Rajesh U Patel, Sai Drashti Eye Hospital, Bharuch).

Ectopia lentis: Marfan's syndrome (Upward dislocation), Homocystinuria (Downward dislocation), Weill Marchesani Syndrome(National Organisation For Rare Disorders)(short stature, ectopia lentis, myopia, microspherophakia, PDA, Pulmonary stenosis, thoracic aortic aneurysm etc).

Retina

It is very obvious that most of the retinal changes occurring in cardiovascular diseases are discovered by Fundoscopy.

➤ **Hypertensive retinopathy**

Choroidopathy ⇒ Fibrinoid necrosis of choroidal arteries

⇩ Elschnig's spots: Retinal pigment epithelium (RPE) appears pale

⇩ Siegrist's streak: RPE hyperplasia

⇩ RPE detachments

Macular changes ⇒ Macular star formation(hard exudate)

Optic nerve damage ⇒ Optic disk swelling

Keith-Wagner- Barker classification of hypertensive retinopathy ⇒

Grade I : Constriction of retinal arterioles

Grade II : Grade I + focal narrowing of retinal arterioles + AV nicking

Grade III : Grade II + flame-shaped hemorrhages + cotton-wool spots + hard exudates

Grade IV : Grade III with Papilledema

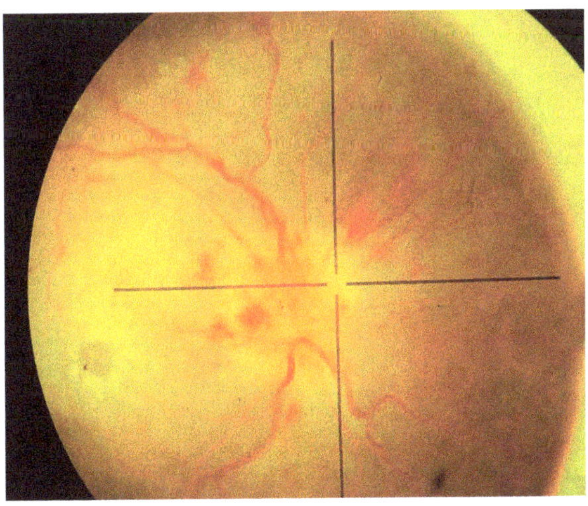

Fig. 1.31: Grade IV hypertensive retinopathy
(Courtesy: Dr. Rajesh U Patel, Sai Drashti Eye Hospital, Bharuch).

- Infective endocarditis (IE):

  Roth spot (2%) ⇒ Retinal hemorrhages with white centre due to accumulation of leucocyte or platelet-fibrin plugs. Other eye findings in IE include conjunctival hemorrhages, chorioretinitis and endophthalmitis.

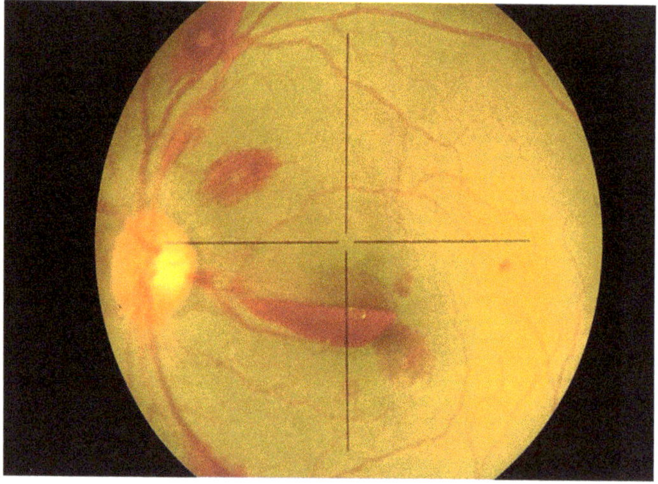

Fig. 1.32: Roth's spots (hemorrhages with pale centre)
(Courtesy: Dr. Rajesh U Patel, Sai Drashti Eye Hospital, Bharuch)

- Coarctation of aorta: Corkscrew-shaped tortuosity of the retinal arteries.
- Retinal embolism:
  - Platelet-fibrin embolism ⇒ Grey-white, mobile material, intravascular in location, occupies a long segment of arteriole before breaking.

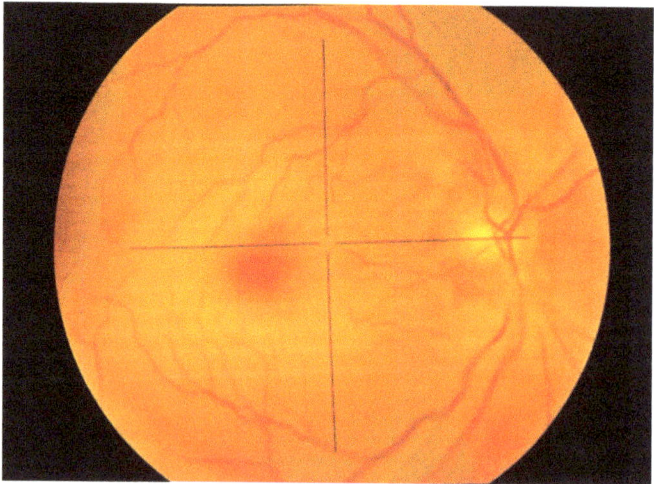

Fig. 1.33: Central retinal artery occlusion following thromboembolism
(Courtesy: Dr. Rajesh U Patel, Sai Drashti Eye Hospital, Bharuch).

- Cholesterol emboli ⇒ Small but multiple, and yellow-white in appearance
- Calcification ⇒ White colored, large sized and commonly located at the proximal retinal arterial branches.
- Common causes of retinal embolism: Carotid artery stenosis, Rheumatic valvular heart diseases, Atrial fibrillation, Diabetes mellitus, Hypertension, Hyperlipidemia, Smoking, H/O IHD.

NOSE

As described above, broad nose is seen in several syndromes like Noonan syndrome, William syndrome, Acromegaly, Down syndrome, Hurler's syndrome, etc.

EARS

→ Earlobe crease (as described above) is an indicator of hyperlipidemia and associated with increased chances of CAD.

→ Low set ears are seen in diseases like Down syndrome, Turner syndrome, Noonan syndrome, William syndrome, Cri du Chat syndrome, Klippel-Feil syndrome, etc (all described above).

→ Low set ear is defined when the helix meets the cranium below an imaginary horizontal line drawn through both the inner canthi of the eyes. (MedicineNet)

LIPS

→ Pallor: Indicates anemia which can lead to high output cardiac failure.

→ Cyanosis: Cyanotic congenital heart diseases.

→ Thick (prominent) lips: William syndrome, Hurler's syndrome, Acromegaly, etc.

→ Thin lips: Fetal alcohol syndrome

→ Long philtrum: William syndrome

→ Small philtrum: Cri du Chat syndrome

→ Angular stomatitis (ulcers at the angle of the mouth): Multivitamin deficiency, congenital syphilis (rhagades).

ORAL CAVITY

→ Improper oral hygiene and gingivitis: Risk factor for developing IE.

→ Gum hyperplasia: Nifedipine use (other drugs like Dilantin and cyclosporine)

→ Petechiae: Infective endocarditis

TEETH

→ Delayed dentition: Hurler's syndrome, cretinism

→ Neonatal teeth: Ellis Van Creveld syndrome

→ Widely spaced teeth: William syndrome, Syphilis, Mucopolysaccharidosis

→ Hutchinson teeth: Peg shaped, widely split, central upper incisors seen in congenital syphilis

→ Mulberry molars: Multicuspid 1st molars seen in congenital syphilis.

TONGUE

→ Pallor: Anemia

→ Cyanosis

→ Fissured tongue: Acromegaly, Trisomy 21

→ Large tongue (macroglossia): Down syndrome, Amyloidosis, Hurler's syndrome, Acromegaly, Hypothyroidism.

PALATE

→ Cleft palate: Syphilis, Velocardiofacial syndrome (retrognathia, long nose, suborbital congestion, hooding of upper eyelids, conotruncal abnormalities)

→ High arched palate: Seen in Marfan syndrome (discussed already).

High arched palate is said to be present if the roof of the palate is not visible when the examiner keeps his eyes at the same level as that of the patient's upper incisors with the mouth wide open.

CYANOSIS

Abnormal bluish discoloration of skin and mucous membranes due to high levels of deoxygenated (reduced) hemoglobin within the superficial dermal capillaries and subpapillary venous plexus.

Best appreciated at sites where epidermis is thin and has abundant blood supply like lips, buccal mucosa, nose, ears, cheeks etc.

Cyanosis occurs if the reduced hemoglobin is > 4 - 6 mg/dl or > 30% of the total Hb and PaO_2 < 85% or due to presence of abnormal Hb pigments in the blood like Methemoglobinemia (>1.5 gm/dl) or Sulfhemoglobinemia (> 0.5 gm/dl).

Cyanosis is of two types

→ Central cyanosis: More worrisome and is generally a late finding in the course of illness.

It requires ↓ PaO_2 or abnormal Hb derivatives.

It usually affects the central structures and mucosae (tongue, oral mucosa and conjunctiva).

→ Peripheral cyanosis: Normal SaO_2 but ↑ extraction of oxygen in the setting of peripheral vasoconstriction and decreased peripheral blood flow.

Usually seen on the cool areas e.g. nose, lips, earlobes and fingertips.

The MC cause of peripheral cyanosis is vasoconstriction due to exposure to cold air or water.

It is important to understand that in cyanosis it is the capillary deoxyhemoglobin that is responsible for the blue discoloration and not the arterial deoxyhemoglobin.

Also, it is the absolute quantity of deoxyhemoglobin that is important for the development of cyanosis and not the relative quantity i.e; the level of SaO_2 at which cyanosis develops depends on the total Hb concentration. Hence an anemic patient with marked arterial desaturation may not develop cyanosis but a polycythemia patient may develop cyanosis at a much higher SaO_2.

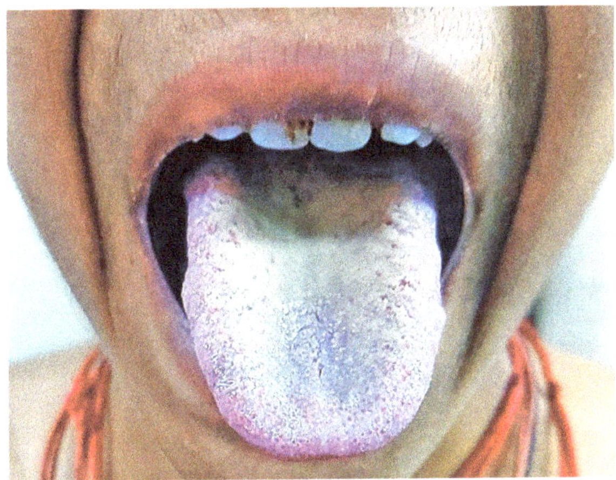

Fig. 1.34: Central cyanosis involving the tongue.

Most of the causes of cyanosis are cardiopulmonary in nature

Also, whenever one finds a case of chronic cyanosis he/she should try to see the most common associated clinical finding........**CLUBBING**, and vice versa.

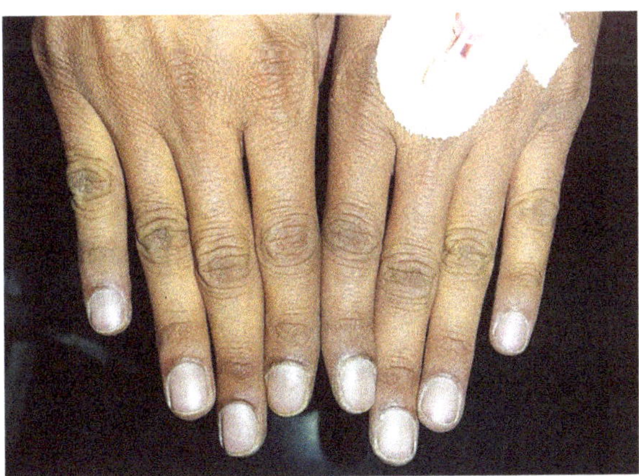

Fig. 1.35: Cyanosis of the nails with clubbing in a case of cyanotic congenital heart disease.

Also, clinically when we are using the bedside pulse oximeter in any case of cyanosis, we should be aware that the pulse oximeter works on the principle of absorption of red and infrared light by the oxy- and deoxygenated Hb, and hence may wrongly show a reduced PaO_2 in peripheral cyanosis (false positive). This can be avoided by doing an Arterial blood gas analysis.

Methemoglobinemia and Sulfhemoglobinemia is suspected if on exposing the patient's blood to 100% O_2 (in a tube) or air, it remains brown.The blood sample from a patient of cyanosis due to ↓ arterial oxygen saturation will turn bright red on exposure to air.

Etiologies of central cyanosis

→ ↓ arterial O_2 saturation ⇒ High altitude, ventilation perfusion mismatch, alveolar hypoventilation, congenital cyanotic heart diseases, Pulmonary AV fistula, low oxygen affinity Hb.

→ Abnormal Hb ⇒ Methemoglobinemia (hereditary, nitrates, sulfonamides), Sulfhemoglobinemia, Carboxyhemoglobinemia (chocolate cyanosis).

Causes of peripheral cyanosis

→ ↓CO (LVF or Shock)

→ Exposure to cold

→ Peripheral vascular diseases (arterial and venous)

→ All etiologies of central cyanosis can also cause peripheral cyanosis.

NOTE

Finger cyanosis > Toe cyanosis ⇒ Complete TGA with either a preductal coarctation or complete interruption of the aortic arch and a reversed shunt through a PDA.

Right hand cyanosis > Left hand cyanosis ⇒ Preductal coarctation of the aorta.

Equal cyanosis of both hands ⇒ Postductal coarctation.

Toe cyanosis > Finger cyanosis ⇒ PDA with Eisenmenger's syndrome.

NECK

Just like any other disease, neck examination is an important part of evaluating any cardiovascular disease. As described above, there are a number of syndromes and diseases that have some neck findings and cardiovascular manifestations as well.

Webbed neck

→ Noonan syndrome

→ Turner's syndrome

Short neck

Short neck is found in a number of syndromes that have CVS components as well (described earlier).

Some of these syndromes are Noonan syndrome, Turner's syndrome, Klippel-Feil syndrome, Mucopolysaccharidoses.

The Bird's Index is used to detect short necks.

Bird's Index is the ratio between height and distance between external occipital protuberance to the spinous process of C7 vertebra.

Normal < 12.8; Short Neck ≥ 13.6

Low Hairline

Defined when the posterior hairline level is below the level of the spinous process of the C5 vertebra.

Seen in Turner's syndrome, Noonan syndrome, Klippel-Feil syndrome.

Abnormal neck swelling

Look for thyroid swelling (hyper- or hypothyroidism), Lymph node swelling (tuberculosis, syphilis, etc), parotid swelling in viral infections like mumps which can affect the heart leading to myocarditis.

SPINE

Spine is one body part that is least sought for when examining a patient with CVS perspective.

But there are a number of syndromes with spinal abnormalities that have cardiovascular defects as well.

Marfan syndrome: Kyphoscoliosis

Ankylosing spondylitis: Aortic insufficiency, aortitis of asc. aorta, AV blocks, MR (less common)

Straight back syndrome (SBS): Loss of thoracic kyphosis → reduced AP diameter of the chest → compression or "pancaking" of the heart and great vessels so as to appear enlarged.

CVS findings in SBS include ⇒ Pulmonary ejection murmur, left parasternal systolic impulse, loud and delayed TV closure sound, exaggerated inspiratory splitting of S2, rSr' pattern in V1 or aVR, prominence of pulmonary arteries on radiology, and cardiomegaly.

All these features of SBS mimic clinical features of atrial septal defect(ASD).

SKIN

The importance of skin changes has been known since the times of Hippocrates. These findings include changes in skin color and texture and also changes occurring in the digits.

Cyanosis: Discussed in detail earlier.

Flushing

- → Carcinoid syndrome leading to flushing of the face, neck and chest due to serotonin production. It is associated with fibrotic tricuspid stenosis and regurgitation as well as pulmonary stenosis.
- → Pheochromocytoma ⇒ episodic flushing of face and forehead ⇒ associated with hypertension.
- → Sipple's syndrome ⇒ generalised flushing due to prostaglandin and serotonin.
- → Severe aortic regurgitation ⇒ Flushing of the nail beds in synchrony with the heart beats (Quincke sign).

Erythremia

Flushing plus cyanosis in the same patient.

Seen in Polycythemia.

Also called 'Ruddy' complexion.

Usually seen in tongue, conjunctiva, nose, lips, earlobes, fingertips and toe - tips.

Erythema

Facial erythema + cyanotic hue + edema of the face + non-pulsatile engorged neck and chest veins is seen in SVC obstruction.

Texture of the skin

- → Dry, coarse skin: Myxedema
- → Smooth, fine skin: Hyperthyroidism
- → Thick skin: Acromegaly
- → Waxy skin with 'Pinch purpura' (skin becomes hemorrhagic when rubbed): - Amyloidosis (associated with cardiomyopathy and postural hypotension due to autonomic neuropathy).
- → Lax skin with hyperextensible joints: - Marfan syndrome, Ehlers-Danlos syndrome.
- → Looseness of the skin with pendulous folds: - Cutis laxa(associated with dilatation and/ or rupture of the aorta).
- → Yellow and lax skin over the axilla: - Pseudoxanthoma elasticum(associated with claudication and angina pectoris, and MVP).
- → Atrophic skin: - Werner's syndrome (associated with premature CAD).

Xanthomatosis

Deposition of lipids underneath the skin, tendons and fascia.

Xanthomas are indicative of premature atherosclerosis and hyperlipidemia.

Hence, searching for cutaneous xanthomas is very important especially when the patient of CAD is young.

Xanthomas can be classified into various types: - plane, tendinous, palmar, tuberous, eruptive.

→ Xanthoma planum (Xanthelasma): Seen above the inner canthus of the eye commonly. Frequently seen in type II and sometimes in type III hyperlipoproteinemia. It is also common in diabetes.

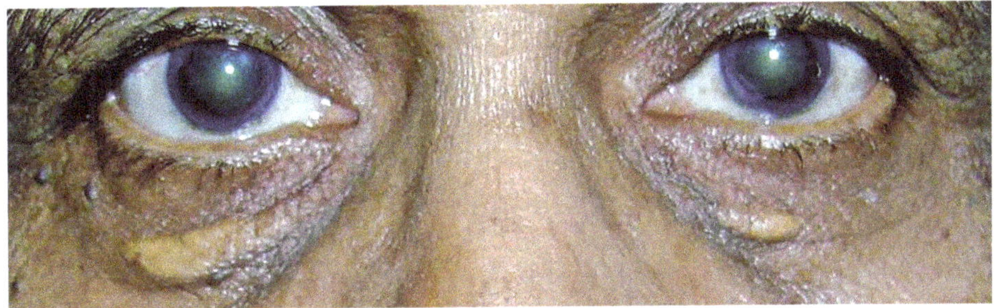

Fig. 1.36: Xanthelasma (Courtesy: Dr. Rajesh U Patel, Sai Drashti Eye Hospital, Bharuch).

→ Tendinous xanthoma: Commonly found in achilles tendon(earliest) and also over the extensor tendons of the hands and feet. They almost invariably indicate hyperlipoproteinemia of long duration and commonly found in familial type IIa hyperlipoproteinemia.

→ Xanthoma striatum palmare: Seen on the creases of the hands. Commonly seen in Type III hyperlipoproteinemia, but can also be seen in obstructive liver disorders.

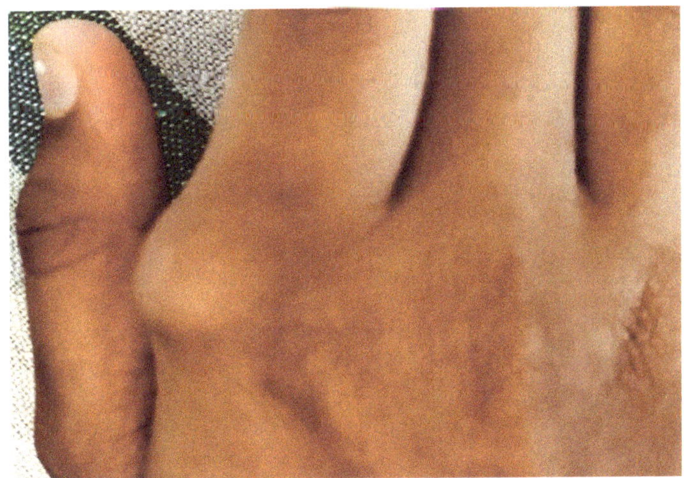

Fig. 1.37: Tendinous xanthoma (Courtesy: Dr. Sriranga R).

→ Tuberous xanthoma: Painless tumors seen over extensor aspects of the elbows, knees and the buttocks. It occurs with type II and type III hyperlipoproteinemia. Somewhat similar "tuberoeruptive" lesions appear with types III and IV.

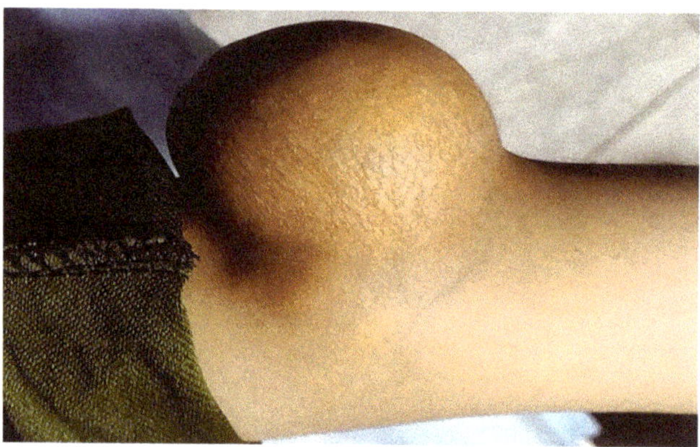

Fig. 1.38: Tuberous xanthoma on the knee (Courtesy: Dr. Sriranga R).

→ Eruptive xanthoma: Yellow papules on the buttocks, abdomen and extremities. They indicate an abrupt rise of serum triglycerides to high levels. This is commonly seen with uncontrolled diabetes mellitus, and type I or V hyperlipoproteinemia.

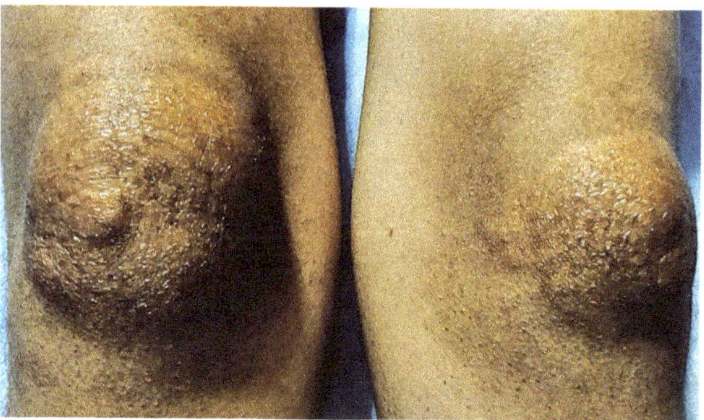

Fig. 1.39: Tendinous xanthoma (Courtesy: Dr. Sriranga R).

Fredrickson classification of hyperlipoproteinemia

Hyperlipo-proteinemia	Other name	↑Lipoprotein	Symptoms
Type I	Familial hyperchylomicronemia	Chylomicrons	Acute pancreatitis, lipemia retinalis, eruptive skin xanthomas, hepatosplenomegaly, Insulin dependent DM, Dysglobulinemia , Autoimmune hyperlipoproteinemia

(Continued)

Hyperlipo-proteinemia	Other name	↑Lipoprotein	Symptoms
Type IIa	Familial hypercholesterolemia	LDL	Xanthelasma, arcus senilis, tendon xanthomas, Hypothyroidism, Nephrotic syndrome, Dysglobulinemia, Familial IHD
Type IIb	Familial combined hyperlipidemia	LDL and VLDL	
Type III	Familial dysbetalipoproteinemia	IDL	Tuberoeruptive xanthomas, Xanthoma striatum palmare, Autoimmune hyperlipoproteinemia
Type IV	Familial hypertriglyceridemia	VLDL	Pancreatitis, Diabetes mellitus, Familial IHD, Hypothyroidism, Nephrotic syndrome, Dysglobulinemia, Autoimmune hyperlipoproteinemia
Type V	Hyperbetalipoprotein-emia and Chylomi-cronemia	VLDL and chylomicrons	Insulin dependent DM , Nephrotic syndrome , Pancreatitis, Dysglobulinemia, Autoimmune hyperlipoproteinemia

Tophi

Occurs due to deposition of uric acid crystals (monosodium urate) in the subcutaneous tissue in gout.

Gout plus hyperuricemia → minor risk factors for CAD.

Tophi very common on the great toe, helix of ear, prepatellar bursa, and olecranon.

Foci of Infective endocarditis

→ Janeway lesions: Papulo-nodular non-tender lesions mostly located on the palms and soles.

› Osler's nodes: Tender, tiny subcutaneous nodules on the fingertips due to immune reaction and micro embolisation of infective materials from the heart valves.

→ Splinter hemorrhages: Commonly found underneath the nails. They are dark red colored, linear streaks.

Foci of peripheral vascular disease

Dry, shiny skin with loss of hair and poor nails and frequently tender ulcers.

Scars

Patients of CAD who have undergone cardiac bypass surgery would have scar marks on the chest and distal part of the medial aspect of the leg from where the long saphenous vein is taken as a graft.

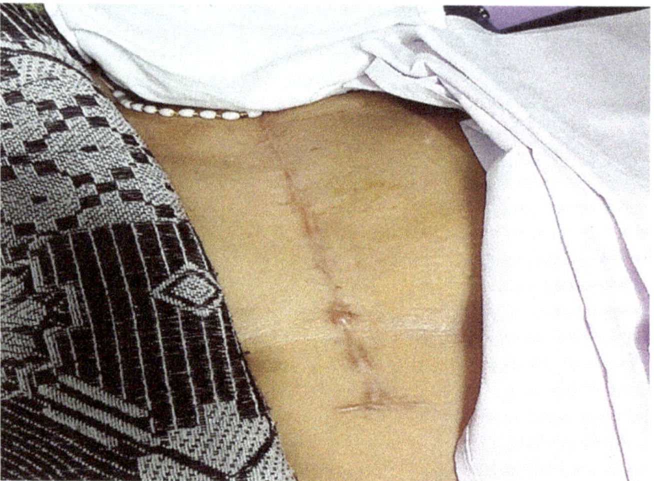

Fig. 1.40: CABG scar mark on the chest.

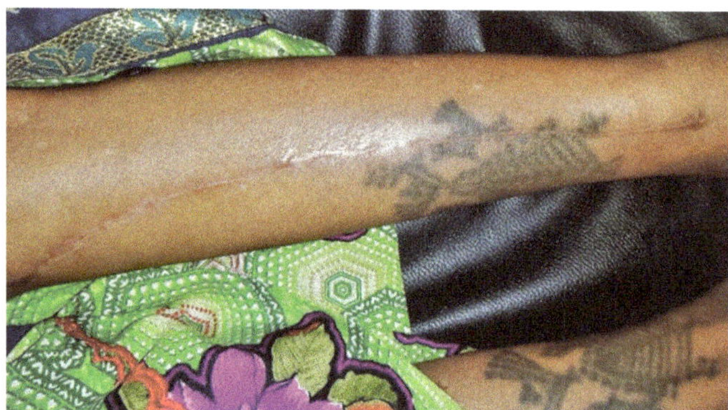

Fig. 1.41: Great saphenous vein graft scar on the medial aspect of the leg in CABG.

Peripheral emboli

Patients with advanced atherosclerosis involving the abdominal aorta may have cholesterol emboli to the lower limbs leading to pain in the legs and down under.

The skin may develop induration, livedo reticularis, and ulceration.

The diagnosis requires deep skin and muscle biopsy.

Foci of atrial myxomas

MC primary tumor of the heart.

Skin findings may include Raynaud's phenomenon, splinter hemorrhages, non-blanching erythema, tender finger pads, etc.

NAME syndrome ⇒ Nevi, Atrial myxoma, Myxoid neurofibromas, Ephelides

LAMB syndrome ⇒ Lentigines, Atrial and Mucocutaneous myxomas, Blue nevi.

Foci of Rheumatic fever

→ Subcutaneous nodules: Freely mobile and painless firm nodules, commonly found over extensor surfaces of fingers and toes and flexor surfaces of the wrist and ankle.

Usually lasts for only 1-2 weeks.

→ Erythema marginatum: Characteristic of Rheumatic fever.

Occurs in 10-25% of the cases.

Nonpruritic macular rash with erythematous and serpiginous border, about 0.5 cm in diameter, and usually located over the trunk and inner aspect of the proximal parts of the limbs.

It is usually accentuated after a hot water bath.

Skin Pigmentation

→ Hemochromatosis: Diffuse slate grey or bronzed appearance of the skin mainly the face, neck, and distal parts of the extremities.

It may lead to a restrictive or dilated cardiomyopathy.

→ Amiodarone toxicity: Blue gray dermal melanosis of the face, especially at the sun exposed areas.

The toxic dose for this manifestation is supposed to be around 600 mg/day for 2 years.

May take several months to resolve after stoppage of the drug due to its long half life.

→ Alkaptonuria: Also called Ochronosis.

Defect in tyrosine metabolism.

Homogentisic acid deposited in skin, joints, ear, and mitral and aortic valves.

Skin over the ears gradually darkens.

Fingernails - blue-gray discoloration.

Most significant cardiac lesion associated - Aortic stenosis.

Multiple Lentigines

Search for features of LEOPARD syndrome (described earlier).

Sarcoidosis

→ Pruritic red papules - eyes, nose, and mouth.

→ Purple plaques, bulky nose, thick cheeks, and thick ears known as 'lupus pernio'.

→ Erythema nodosum - red nodules on the legs.

Cardiovascular manifestations include: heart failure, ventricular tachycardia, complete heart block, and cor pulmonale.

Cardiovascular drugs causing skin changes

→ Warfarin: Skin necrosis

→ Anticoagulants: Bruising of the flanks (Grey Turner's sign) or around the umbilicus (Cullen's sign).

Pallor

→ Anemia

→ Myxedema

Café au lait spots (macules)

If multiple and > 1.5 cm in diameter → may indicate Neurofibromatosis.

Other lesions could be neurofibromas and freckles in the axilla and inguinal region.

Café au lait spots (macules) are common over back and chest.

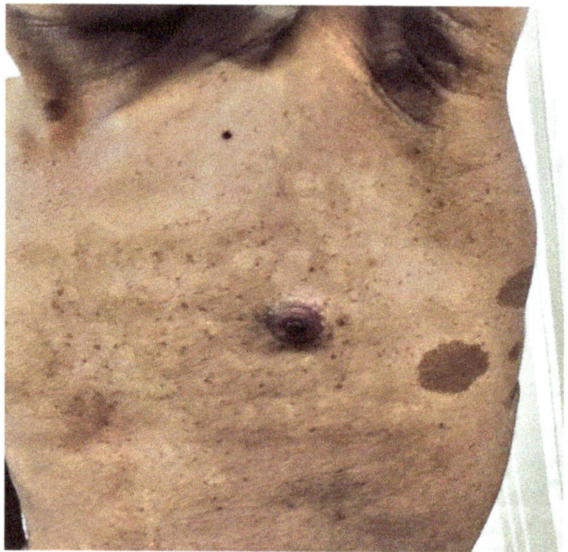

Fig. 1.42: Café au lait macules (Courtesy: Dr Som Lakhani, MD Skin and VD).

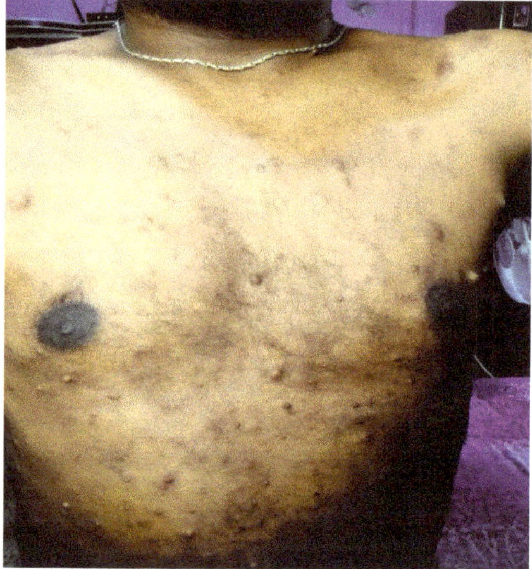

Fig. 1.43: Neurofibromas.

CVS manifestation of neurofibromatosis includes hypertension due to renal artery stenosis or pheochromocytoma.

UPPER LIMBS

A number of abnormalities occur in the upper limbs in a number of diseases that have cardiovascular manifestations also.

These defects include abnormalities of the digits, abnormalities of the nails, Raynaud's phenomenon, etc.

Abnormalities of the digits

→ Arachnodactyly: Also called 'Spider fingers'.

Fingers and toes abnormally longer and slender when compared to the palm of the hand and foot arch.

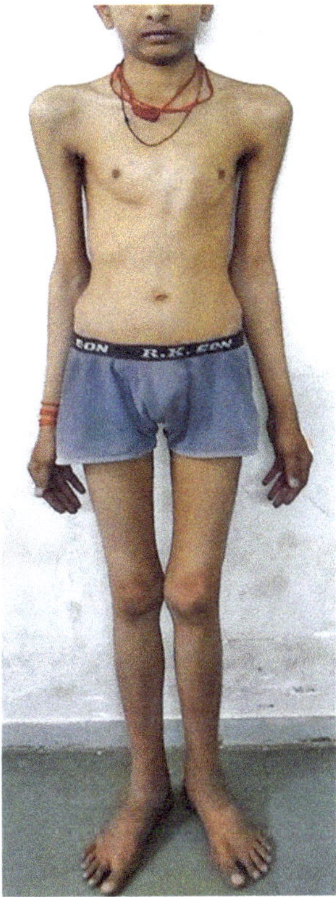

Fig. 1.44

Seen in Marfan's syndrome and Ehlers-Danlos syndrome.

Metacarpal Index(MCI) = Average length of the four metacarpals/Average midwidth of the four metacarpals.

Normal MCI ⇒ 5.4-7.9

MCI > 8.4 ⇒ Marfan's syndrome

→ Polydactyly: Ellis van creveld syndrome and laurence-Moon-Biedl syndrome (discussed earlier).

→ Clinodactyly: (MedicineNet)

Curving of the 5th finger towards the 4th finger.

Also called '5th finger clinodactyly'.

Commonly seen in Down syndrome and Klinefelter (XXY) syndrome.

→ Brachydactyly: Shortened fingers and short hand.

Seen in Down's syndrome, Noonan syndrome, Turner syndrome.

Down's syndrome patients also show Simian crease (single transverse palmar crease).

→ Syndactyly: Failure of the adjacent fingers and/or toes during limb development and hence they are webbed.

→ Sclerodactyly: Tightening of skin on the dorsum of the hand with flexion contractures of the IP joints leading to claw hand deformity.

There is also focal finger tip skin necrosis called 'Rat bite necrosis'.

→ Long 4th finger: Turner syndrome

→ Small 5th finger: Down's syndrome, Kabuki syndrome.

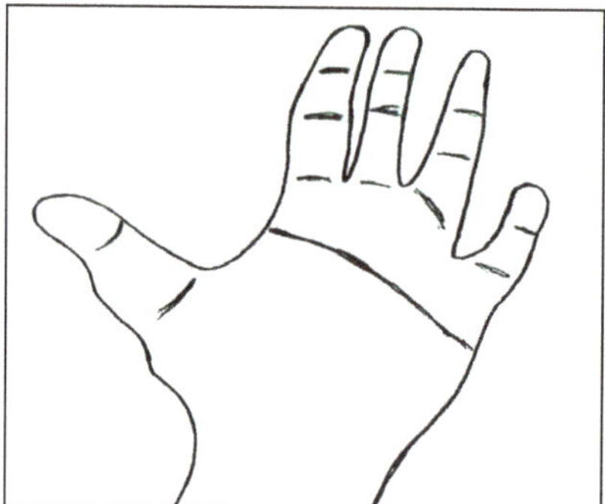

Fig. 1.45: Small 5th finger with single crease in Down's syndrome.

→ Long 1st proximal phalanx (Fingerized thumb) or missing thumb or an extra digit: Holt-Oram syndrome (associated with secundum ASD).

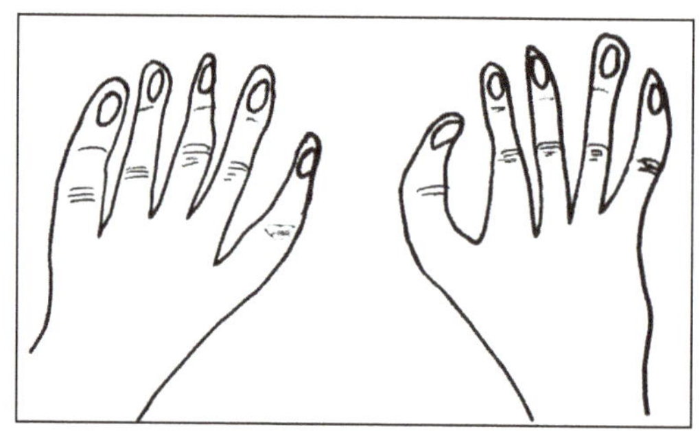

Fig. 1.46: Fingerized thumb in Holt-Oram syndrome.

→ Spade shaped hands: Acromegaly

Palmar erythema

Although a sign more specific for liver failure, there are some diseases that have cardiovascular components in addition to palmar erythema e.g.; thyrotoxicosis, hemochromatosis, diabetes, smoking, rheumatoid arthritis, etc.

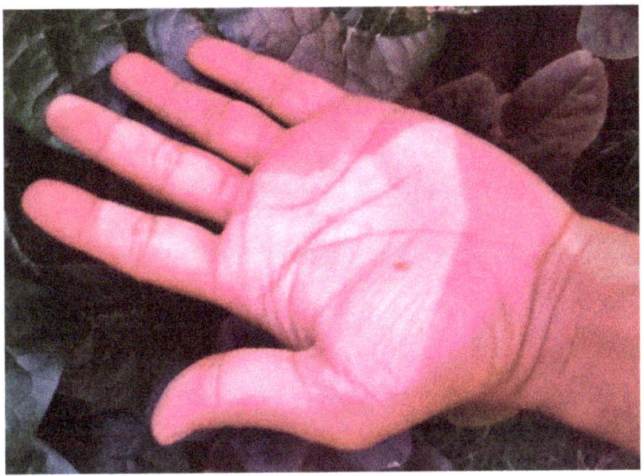

Fig. 1.47: Palmar erythema.

Tremor of the outstretched hands: Thyrotoxicosis

Raynaud's phenomenon

Spasm of arteries cause episodes of reduced blood flow.The episodes result in the affected part turning white and then blue. Fingers affected > than the toes.

Seen in SLE, Scleroderma, CREST syndrome.

SLE patients also show red plaques over the dorsum of the hands.

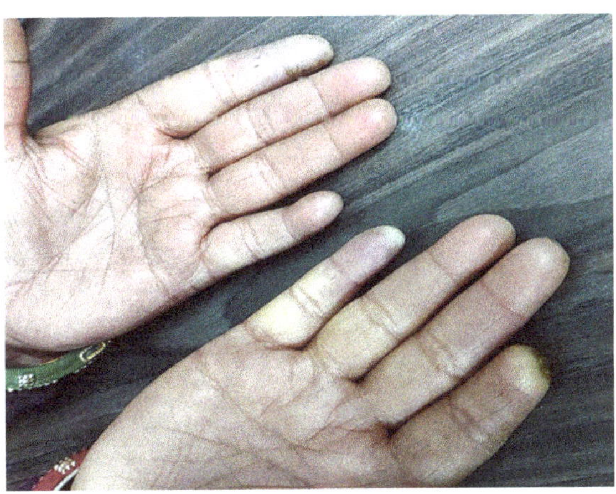

Fig. 1.48: Raynaud's phenomenon
(note the paleness of right ring and little fingers with autoamputation of the index finger in scleroderma) .

Gottron's papules

Found over the knuckles in Dermatomyositis.

Also called Violaceous papules.

CVS manifestations in Dermatomyositis include CHF, pericarditis and heart block.

Edema of the upper limbs: SVC obstruction

Swollen arm with distended veins over them: Subclavian vein thrombosis

Locomotor brachialis

Prominent pulsation of a usually tortuous brachial artery.

Usually considered as a sign of premature atherosclerosis or dyslipidemia but also a peripheral sign of severe AR.

Scar mark

For example radial artery harvesting for CABG graft.

NAILS

Nails are examined for cyanosis, clubbing, subungual hemorrhages, color changes, etc.

Cyanosis, Splinter hemorrhages: Discussed earlier.

Capillary pulsations: When a gentle pressure is applied on the nail, rhythmic nail bed flushing can be seen synchronous with heart beats in severe aortic regurgitation (Quincke's sign).

Muehrcke's nails

Firstly described by Dr. Robert Muehrcke in 1956.

It is an example of apparent leukonychia where there are static white discoloration bands secondary to nail bed pathology.

In true leukonychia there is a white band in the nail matrix secondary to injury that moves with nail growth.

Causes include ⇒ Hypoalbuminemia, severe malnutrition, liver diseases, renal insufficiency, pellagra and chemotherapy drugs (most frequently doxorubicin and cyclophosphamide).

Platonychia (flat, broad nail)

Acromegaly

White nails (Terry nails)

White-colored proximal half and normal distal half.

Seen in CHF, liver cirrhosis, and adult-onset diabetes mellitus.

Blue–gray nails

Seen in hemochromatosis, Wilson's disease, and ochronosis.

Black nails

Cushing's syndrome (hypertension).

Plummer's nails (Onycholysis)

Seen in hyperthyroidism, trauma, psoriasis or syphilis.

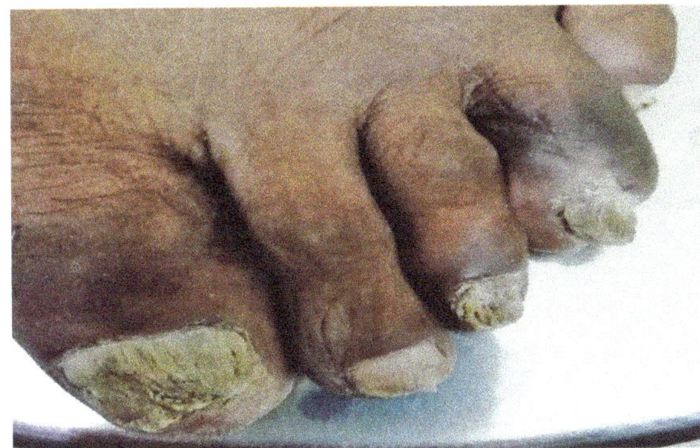

Fig. 1.49: Onycholysis (Courtesy: Dr. Som Lakhani, MD Skin and VD).

Koilonychia (Spoon shaped nails)

Seen in Iron deficiency anemia which may lead to high output cardiac failure.

Also, pallor of the nail bed is seen in anemia.

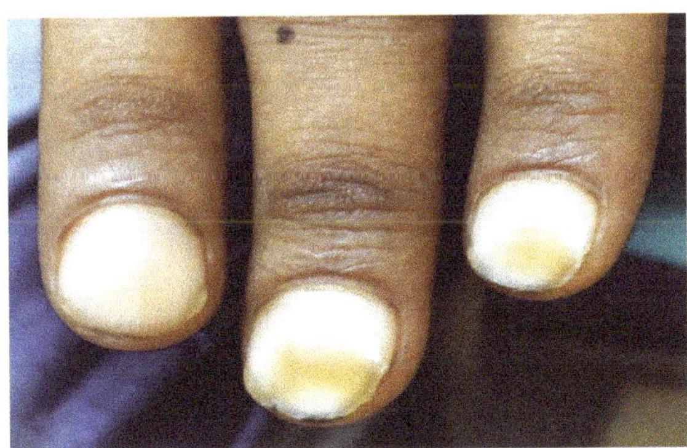

Fig. 1.50: Koilonychia (Courtesy: Dr.Som Lakhani, MD Skin and VD).

Lindsay nails ("half-and-half nails")

Proximal half is normal and distal half-nail is brown.

Common in renal failure patients with uremia.

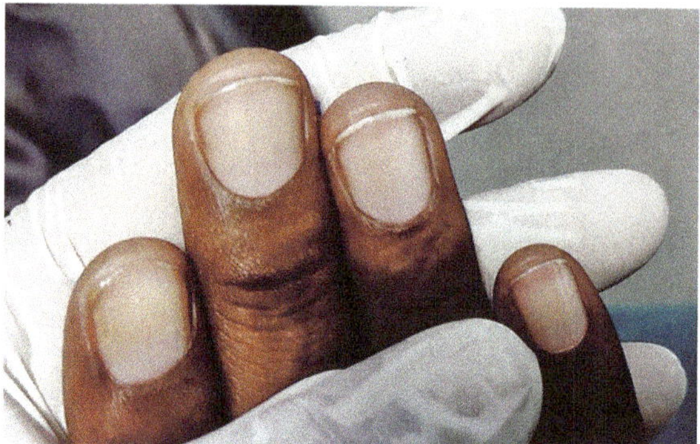

Fig. 1.51: Lindsay nails.

Beau's lines

White depression lines due to direct damage to the nail matrix by antimitotic drugs (commonly taxanes).

The line width is directly related to the severity and chronicity of the underlying disease.

Mees' lines

These are true leukonychia.

Causes include arsenic trioxide poisoning, leprosy, tuberculosis, malaria, herpes zoster, CO, thallium, and chronic fluoride poisoning (fluorosis), infections , Hodgkin lymphoma, acute myeloid leukemia, and chemotherapy.

Digital compression fails to fade these lesions (unlike Muehrcke's lines), and they keep on moving along the nail growth.

Clubbing

Oldest clinical sign in Medicine.

Bulbous uniform swelling of the terminal phalanx.

Loss of the angle between the nail and the nail bed which is present normally.

Other names for clubbing ⇒ Hippocratic nails, Trommelschlegelfinger, watch-glass nails, and serpent head nails.

Usually acquired and often reversible.

Usually painless, but can be painful if there is hypertrophic osteoarthropathy (HOA) which is periostitis of the long bones, joint pain and clubbing.

Clubbing is due to a pulmonary cause in 75-80%, cardiovascular cause in 10-15%, GIT/hepatic cause in 5-10% and miscellaneous in 5-10%.

2% of healthy people can have clubbing.

Pathophysiological theories of clubbing:

- Vascular endothelial growth factor produced in various malignancies and hypoxia causes hyperplasia of vasculature, edema and osteoblast proliferation causing clubbing.
- Megakaryocytes from the bone marrow break down into platelet clumps and get deposited at the fingertips under various circumstances and release platelet derived growth factors that cause hypertrophy of connective tissues leading to clubbing.
- A neural mechanism with vagal activation leading to increased blood flow and clubbing has also been postulated.
- Growth hormone has also been implicated as a causative factor in clubbing.

Thumb and the forefingers are usually the first places where clubbing develops.

Floating nail sign ⇒ Normally when pressure is applied to the root of the nail plate, there is no movement. But in clubbing this pressure produces movement of the nail plate towards the bone.

Profile sign ⇒ Increase in the Lovibond's angle i.e; angle between the nail plate and skin over the proximal part of the distal phalanx. Normal Lovibond's angle is < 160^0

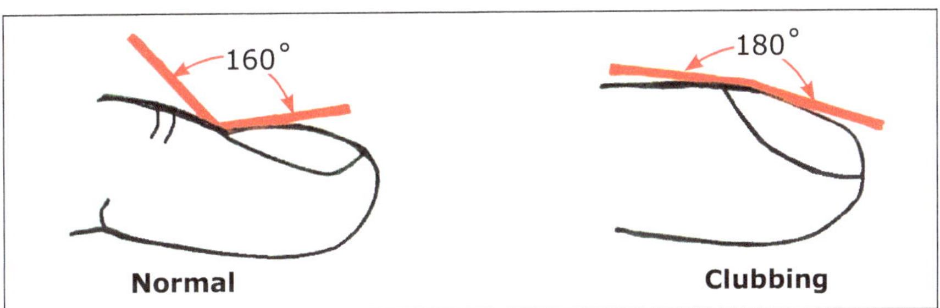

Fig. 1.52

Profile sign is the first sign to occur in clubbing.

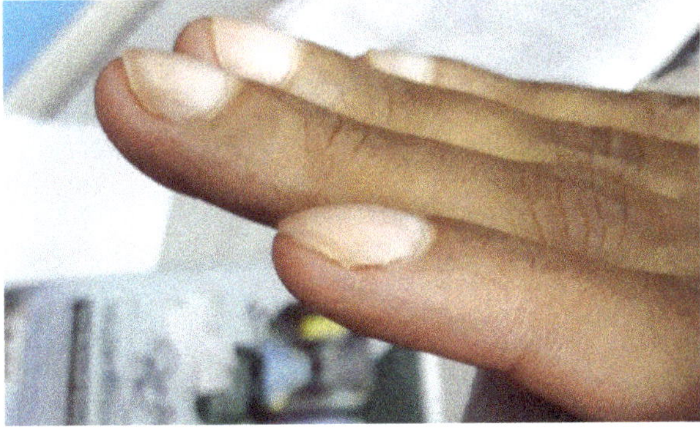

Fig. 1.53

Schamroth sign ⇒ When the dorsum of the distal phalanges of the thumbs (or any other finger) of both hands are placed approximated to each other, a small diamond shaped gap is observed due to the Lovibond's angle. This gap disappears in clubbing due to obliteration of the angle.

Schamroth sign is useful to distinguish clubbing from pseudoclubbing.

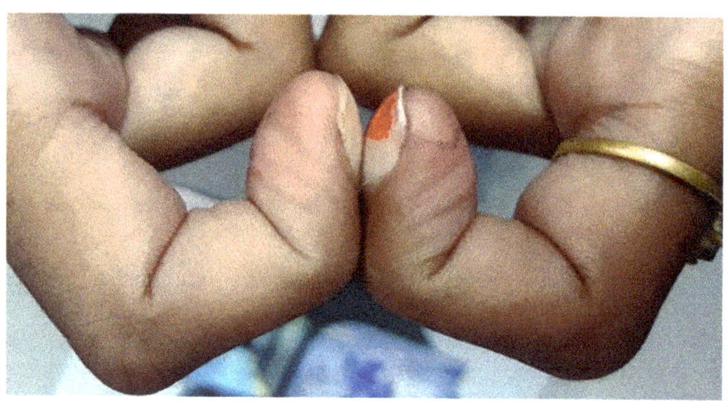

Fig. 1.54: Schamroth sign.

Schamroth sign

Grades of clubbing:

Grade I → Obliteration of the nail bed angle and positive fluctuation test

Grade II → Grade I plus ↑ AP and transverse diameter of the nails.

Grade III → Grade II plus ↑ in pulp tissue (Parrot beak/Drumstick appearance)

Grade IV → Grade III plus hypertrophic osteoarthropathy.

Causes of clubbing:

Pulmonary ⇒ Bronchogenic carcinoma, mesothelioma, thymoma, metastatic CA, lung abscess, chronic empyema, pneumoconiosis, cystic fibrosis, chronic pneumonitis, bronchiectasis etc.

Cardiovascular causes ⇒ Cyanotic congenital heart diseases, subacute bacterial endocarditis, atrial myxoma, pulmonary AV fistula, cor pulmonale, chronic congestive heart failure.

GIT and hepatic causes ⇒ Cirrhosis of liver, ulcerative colitis, Crohn's disease, gut malignancies.

Miscellaneous causes ⇒ Hyperthyroidism, hyperparathyroidism, pregnancy, Syphilis, Acromegaly, syringomyelia, Arsenic, Mercury, Beryllium, Silica, Phosphorus, Alcohol, chronic laxative abuse.

It is worthy to note that Tuberculosis (TB) alone does not usually cause clubbing. However, cavitating TB or TB with HIV co infection or TB with bronchiectasis can produce clubbing.

Causes of unilateral clubbing:

→ Aneurysm of the aorta, subclavian artery or axillary artery

→ Brachial AV fistula

→ Pancoast tumor

→ Erythromelalgia

→ Hemiplegia

→ Lymphangitis

→ Subungual fibroma

Causes of unidigital clubbing:

→ Trauma

→ Tophaceous gout

→ Sarcoidosis

→ Injury to the Median nerve

Causes of pseudoclubbing:

Single digit→ Pseudocyst, subungual fibroma, osteoid osteoma.

Generalised→ Hansen's disease, Leukemia, Hyperparathyroidism and any other condition causing acro-osteolysis.

Treatment of clubbing needs treatment of the cause that usually leads to complete resolution.

A new onset clubbing in any patient with COPD indicates the onset of bronchogenic carcinoma, provided that we have ruled out lung abscess and bronchiectasis.

Congenital cyanotic heart disease with clubbing usually indicates a reversal of the shunt.

LOWER LIMBS

Pes cavus

Unusually high plantar arch.

The foot maintains a distinctly hollow form when it is bearing weight.

Friedreich's ataxia is characterized by the triad of Pes cavus, nystagmus and sensory ataxia.

Cardiomyopathy is frequently associated with this type of ataxia.

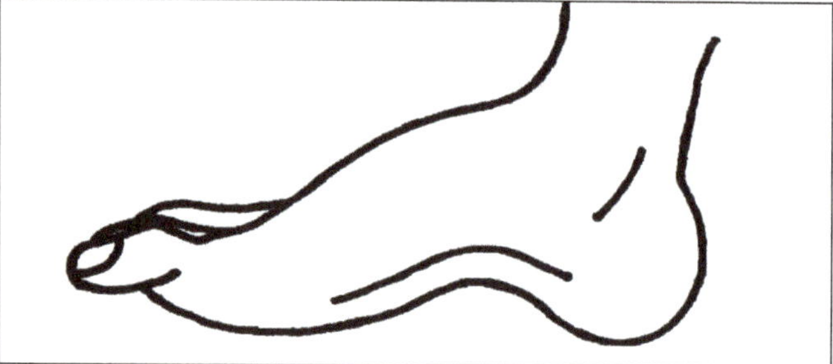

Fig. 1.55: Pes cavus.

Pes planus

Also called 'Flat feet'.

Loss of the medial longitudinal arch of the foot where it contacts the ground.

Commonly seen in Rheumatoid arthritis, Down's syndrome, Marfan syndrome and Ehlers-Danlos syndrome.

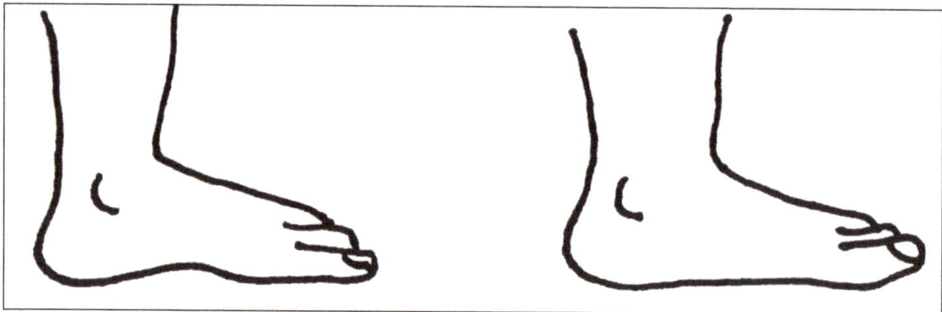

Fig. 1.56: Pes planus.

Rocker bottom feet

Excessive posteriorly protruding heel is seen in Edward's syndrome.

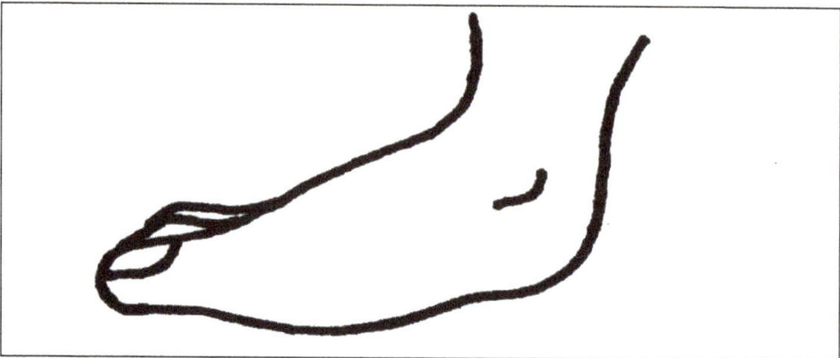

Fig. 1.57: Rocker bottom feet.

Saber shin

Sharp anterior bowing, or convexity, of the tibia.

Seen in syphilis, yaws, Paget's disease of bone, vitamin D deficiency or Weismann-Netter–Stuhl syndrome, osteomalacia.

Knock knees

Also called Genu valgum.

Seen in Ellis-van Creveld syndrome, and Laurence-Moon-Biedl syndrome.

Rare cases of Laurence-Moon-Biedl syndrome have also shown Genu varum with tibia vara.

Hyperextensible (lax) joints

Seen in Marfan syndrome and Ehlers-Danlos syndrome.

ARTHRITIS

Migratory polyarthritis

Rapid onset swelling and pain in one or two joints with resolution within a few days.

Usually asymmetric in location.

Seen in gonococcal arthritis, rheumatic fever, sarcoidosis, SLE, Lyme disease, bacterial endocarditis, and Whipple's disease.

Intermittent arthritis

Symptoms for a few days to months and then complete resolution followed by reappearance of symptoms.

Usually seen in gout (as stated earlier, gout is a minor risk factor for CAD).

Rheumatic fever arthritis (ARF)

→ Migratory polyarthritis

→ Involves mainly the large joints at multiple sites e.g; knees, elbows, ankles, wrists

→ Pain subsides within 2-4 weeks without any residual deformity

→ Pain responds dramatically to salicylates within 24-48 hours

→ Rheumatic fever causes carditis (which is also one of the components of the **Jones criteria#**)

Poststreptococcal reactive arthritis (PSA)

→ The diagnosis of PSA is considered when a patient has similar clinical features of ARF but does not satisfy the Jones criteria for ARF and also does not respond to salicylates.

→ PSA begins sooner (approximately 10 days) after streptococcal infection than does ARF (approximately 21 days).

→ The bone pain is persistent and also involves the smaller joints.

→ Deformity may occur.

Gout

→ Gout and hyperuricemia is a minor risk factor for CAD.

→ Hyperuricemia has also been found to be associated with atrial fibrillation and heart failure.

→ Gouty arthritis (tophi containing monosodium urate) usually affects one joint, most commonly the metatarsophalangeal joint of the great toe and is aggravated by taking alcohol.

→ Tophi can also form at the helix of the ear.

Rheumatoid arthritis

→ Joint stiffness in the early morning lasting > 1 h that eases with physical activity

→ Involves the small joints of the hands and feet

→ May be monoarticular, oligoarticular (≤ 4 joints) or polyarticular (> 5 joints)

→ Symmetric distribution

→ Involves the wrists, metacarpophalangeal (MCP), and proximal interphalangeal (PIP) joints sparing the distal interphalangeal (DIP) joints

→ Swan neck deformity: Hyperextension of PIP with flexion of DIP joint.

→ Boutonniere deformity: Flexion of PIP joint with hyperextension of DIP joint.

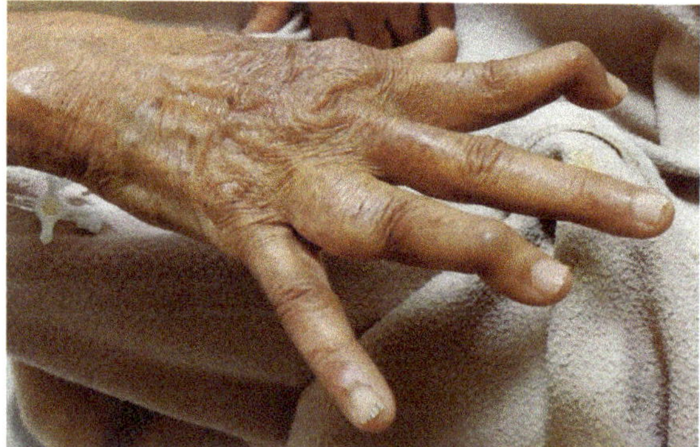

Fig. 1.58: Swan neck deformity in RA (Courtesy: Dr. Chetan Chauhan, Hriday Clinic, Baroda).

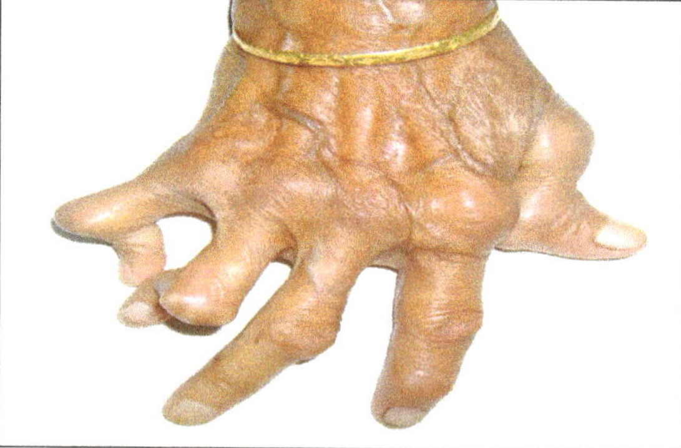

Fig. 1.59: Boutonniere deformity (Courtesy: Dr. Rajesh U Patel, Sai Drashti Eye Hospital, Bharuch).

→ Z- line deformity: Subluxation of first MCP joint with hyperextension of first IP joint.

→ Cardiovascular complications in Rheumatoid arthritis are: pericarditis, IHD, myocarditis, cardiomyopathy, arrhythmia, MR.

 # Revised Jones criteria for Acute Rheumatic Fever

➤ Major criteria: carditis, chorea, arthritis (polyarthritis, or polyarthralgia), Erythema marginatum, and subcutaneous nodules

➤ Minor criteria: fever (≥ 38.5° F), ESR ≥ 30 mm at 1 hour and/or CRP ≥ 3.0 mg/dl, and PR interval prolongation (unless carditis is present)

2 major criteria, or 1 major plus 2 minor criteria means a positive evidence of ARF.

PEDAL EDEMA

Edema is defined as abnormal fluid collection in the interstitial space which is more than the capacity of the physiological lymphatic drainage.

It is the hydrostatic and oncotic pressure gradients across the capillary beds and the lymphatic system that maintains the fluid status of the interstitial space.

Any abnormalities of: -

→ the capillary permeability,

→ the capillary hydrostatic pressure,

→ the capillary oncotic pressure,

→ the lymphatic drainage system,

would lead to the development of pedal edema.

Etiologies of pedal edema based on the above mechanisms are

↑ capillary permeability ⇒ allergy, cellulitis

↑ hydrostatic pressure ⇒ CCF, anemia, renal failure, pregnancy, deep vein thrombosis, compartment syndrome etc.

↓ oncotic pressure ⇒ liver diseases, nephrotic syndrome, protein losing enteropathy, malabsorption syndrome.

Lymphatic obstruction ⇒ tumor, trauma, filariasis, radiation, congenital lymphedema(< 2 years of age), lymphedema precox (females < 35 years of age), lymphedema tarda(> 35 years of age).

Approach to a patient with pedal edema

Uni/Bilateral pedal edema and duration of onset

→ Acute unilateral: DVT, Baker's cyst rupture, compartment syndrome

→ Chronic unilateral: Lymphedema, Pelvic mass, venous insufficiency, reflex sympathetic dystrophy

→ Acute bilateral: DVT, sudden onset CCF

→ Chronic bilateral: Heart failure, drugs, pregnancy, lymphedema, premenstrual edema, kidney diseases, liver diseases, hypothyroidism, anemia, venous insufficiency, etc.

Presence/absence of pain

→ Painful pedal edema: DVT, cellulitis

→ Painless pedal edema: CCF, lymphedema, hypoalbuminemia

Aggravating/relieving factors, appropriate symptoms and history

→ Pedal edema due to cardiac cause (e.g.; CCF) is more during the evening due to upright posture throughout the day and decreases on lying down with a pillow under the feet. Patients who are bedridden can develop edema over the sacral region. There could be h/o associated PND or orthopnea, JVP may be raised, BP higher, cool extremities, S3, chest pain, etc.

→ Pedal edema can occur in renal failure also. But there is H/O periorbital edema that is more in the morning due to lying posture and decreases as the day progresses. It is important to take H/O reduced urine output, hypertension, uremic symptoms, H/O dialysis, childhood diabetes mellitus, etc.

→ Pedal edema due to hepatic cause will usually persist throughout the day with a normal or low JVP, ascites, H/O alcoholism, normal or low BP, features of liver failure (palmar erythema, spider nevi, fetor hepaticus, etc).

→ Idiopathic edema in females usually persists throughout the day in upright posture.

→ Pedal edema in myxedema will be associated with dry skin, bradycardia, sparse hair, hoarse voice,

H/O drug ingestion, trauma and radiation

→ Trauma and radiation can cause cellulitis, compartment syndrome and lymphedema leading to pedal edema.

→ Drugs causing pedal edema are: CCBs, Beta blockers, Corticosteroids, Estrogen, Progesterone, NSAIDs, PPARγ agonists like Pioglitazone.

Pitting vs Non pitting edema

→ Non pitting edema: Myxedema, Pretibial myxedema secondary to Grave's disease, Filariasis(lymphatic obstruction).

However, pitting edema can be seen in the early stages of lymphedema.

→ Most of the other diseases cause pitting pedal edema.

NOTE

To check for pedal edema, just apply firm pressure approximately 1 inch above the medial malleolus with either the thumb or three fingers for about 15 seconds.

It should be "valleys between the hills" if there is pedal edema.

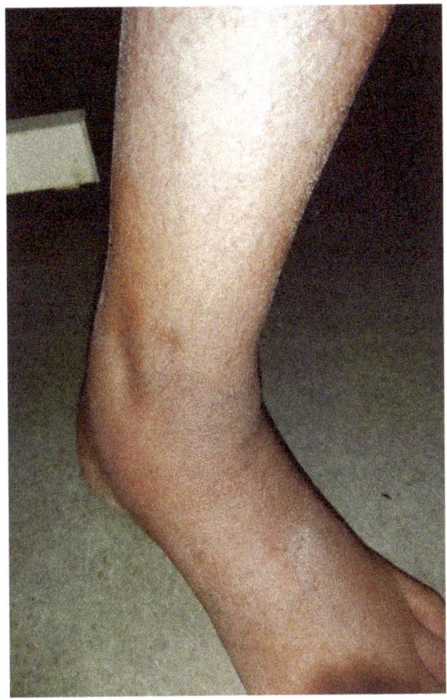

Fig. 1.60: Pitting pedal noted just above the medial malleolus.

References

- Clinical examination in cardiology by B N Vijay Raghawa Rao, 2nd edition.
- Clinical methods in cardiology by B Soma Raju.
- American Family Physician; www.aafp.org/afp; Volume 71, Number 4 • February 15, 2005; Diagnostic Approach to Palpitations by ALLAN V. ABBOTT.
- [Medical news today - "Baldness linked to higher risk of coronary heart disease"......Sarah Glynn on April 4, 2013.]
- Arch Dis Child. 2007 Apr; 92(4): 351-356; Marfan's syndrome and the heart.
- J Pediatr Neurosci. 2010 Jul-Dec; 5(2): 129-131; "Homocystinuria: A rare condition presenting as stroke and megaloblastic anemia".
- J Endocrinol Invest (2017) 40:705-712; Klinefelter syndrome: cardiovascular abnormalities and metabolic disorders.
- Circulation: Genomic and Precision Medicine Volume 11, Issue 10, October 2018; Cardiovascular Health in Turner Syndrome: A Scientific Statement From the American Heart Association.

- Images Paediatr Cardiol. 2001 Apr-Jun; 3(2): 19–30; Clinical manifestations of Noonan syndrome.
- Pediatr Cardiol. 2011 Oct;32(7):977-82. Epub 2011 May 1; Ellis-van Creveld syndrome and congenital heart defects: presentation of an additional 32 cases.
- Orphanet J Rare Dis. 2007; 2: 27.; Ellis-Van Creveld syndrome.
- Journal of Postgraduate Medicine • April 2016 DOI: 10.4103/0022-3859.167730; "FISHed" out the diagnosis: A case of DiGeorge syndrome.
- Korean Circulation Journal http://dx.doi.org/10.4070/kcj.2015.45.5.357 Print ISSN 1738-5520 • On-line ISSN 1738-5555; Genetic Syndromes associated with Congenital Heart Disease.
- Genetics Home Reference; Kabuki syndrome.
- Treat Endocrinol. 2004;3(5):309-18; Cardiac abnormalities in acromegaly. Pathophysiology and implications for management..
- Neuroendocrinology 2010;92(suppl 1):50–54 DOI: 10.1159/000318566; Cardiovascular Disease in Cushing's Syndrome: Heart versus Vasculature.
- British Heart Journal, 1976, 38, 1220-1221 Klippel-Feil syndrome associated with aortic coarctation.
- Indian Pacing Electrophysiol J. 2010; 10(12): 547–550;Kearns Sayre Syndrome (KSS) - A Rare Cause For Cardiac Pacing.
- British Medical Journal;JAN. 28, 1961;CARDIAC LESIONS IN REITER'S DISEASE.
- Journal of Inherited Metabolic Disease; 37,269–276(2014) Mucopolysaccharidosis VI: cardiac involvement and the impact of enzyme replacement therapy.
- Journal of Inherited Metabolic Disease 36, 309–322(2013); Clinical overview and treatment options for non-skeletal manifestations of mucopolysaccharidosis type IVA.
- Am J Cardiol. 2009 Jan 1; 103(1): 64–66;Relation of Corneal Arcus to Cardiovascular Disease (From the Framingham Heart Study Data Set.
- Journal of Dr. D.Y. Patil Vidyapeeth; GUEST EDITORIAL; Year : 2017 | Volume: 10 | Issue: 2 | Page: 118-119; Ocular manifestations of Marfan's syndrome.
- Indian Pediatrics 2002; 39: 97; BrushField spots.
- Am J Dis Child. 1973;126(1):16-18. doi:10.1001/archpedi. 1973. 02110190012003; Congenital Cardiac Disease and the "Cat Eye" Syndrome.
- GeneReviews® [Internet] Adam MP, Ardinger HH, Pagon RA, et al., editors. Seattle (WA): University of Washington, Seattle; 1993-2020;CHARGE Syndrome.
- Comprehensive Vascular and Endovascular Surgery (Second Edition), 2009.
- Medicine Baltimore. 2016 Jul; 95(28): e4119.Published online 2016 Jul 18. doi: 10.1097/MD.0000000000004119;Increased risk of ischemic heart disease among subjects with cataracts.
- The department of clinical neuroscience, section of ophthalmology and vision, St. Erik Eye Hospital Karolinska Institutet, Stockholm, Sweden Congenital Ectopia Lentis - diagnosis and treatment.
- The characteristics of retinal emboli and its association with vascular reperfusion in retinal artery occlusion. Invest Ophthalmol Vis Sci. 2016;57:4589–4598. DOI:10.1167/ iovs.16-19887.
- QJM: An International Journal of Medicine, 2015, 909–910 doi: 10.1093/qjmed/hcv055 Advance Access Publication Date: 11 March 2015 Case report; Classical eye signs in bacterial endocarditis.

- Treasure Island (FL): StatPearls Publishing; 2020 Jan-.Hypertensive Retinopathy.
- Brit. J. Ophthal., 35, 143. Retinal Changes In Coarctation Of The Aorta.
- J Am Dent Assoc. 2009 October; 140(10): 1238–1244. Poor oral hygiene as a risk factor for infective endocarditis- related bacteremia.
- Contemp Clin Dent. 2012 Apr; 3(Suppl1): S55–S59 Oral manifestations of Ellis-van Creveld syndrome)
- Contemp Clin Dent. 2015 Jul-Sep; 6(3): 418–420 Dental management of patient with Williams Syndrome - A case report.
- ScienceDirect; Syphilis;Tobias R. Kollmann, Simon Dobson, in Infectious Diseases of the Fetus and Newborn (Seventh Edition), 2011.
- Int J Pediatr Otorhinolaryngol. 2011 September; 75(9): 1167–1172. doi:10.1016/j.ijporl.2011.06.013. Cleft Palate, Retrognathia and Congenital Heart Disease in VeloCardio-Facial Syndrome: A Phenotype Correlation Study.
- The American College Of Medicine; Division of Critical Care/Department of Anaesthesia, Dalhousie University, Halifax, NS, Canada; Cyanosis.
- Clinical Methods: The History, Physical, and Laboratory Examinations. 3rd edition; Chapter 45 Cyanosis.
- Singapore Med J 1990; Vol 31: 480-485 Cutaneous Manifestations of Cardiac Diseases.
- Bedside Cardiology By Achyut Sarkar.
- Indian Pediatrics Volume31-October1994; Evaluation of Short Neck: New Neck Length Percentiles And Linear Correlations With Height And Sitting Height.
- J Clin Med Res. 2016 Jun; 8(6): 427–430.Published online 2016 May 25. doi: 10.14740/jocmr2488w; Cardiac Involvement in Ankylosing Spondylitis.
- Originally published1 Aug 1965https://doi.org/10.1161/01.CIR.32.2.193 Circulation. 1965; 32:193–203; The Straight Back Syndrome Clinical Cardiovascular Manifestations.
- Singapore Med J 1990; Vol 31: 480-485; Cutaneous Manifestations Of Cardiac Diseases.
- Circulation, Volume XLV, February 1972 World Health Organization Memorandum Classification of Hyperlipidemias and Hyperlipoproteinemias.
- The Art and Science of Cardiac Physical Examination pp 361-395 Local and Systemic Manifestations of Cardiovascular Disease.
- Eur J Hum Genet. 2012 Aug; 20(8): 817–824Syndactyly: phenotypes, genetics and current classification)
- Autops Case Rep. 2018 Jan-Mar; 8(1): e2018014 Muehrcke's lines.
- Transl Pediatr. 2017 Oct; 6(4): 300–312 Dermatologic manifestations of endocrine disorders.
- CHRISMED Journal of Health and Research | Volume 6 | Issue 1 | January-March 2019 Clubbing: The oldest clinical sign in medicine.
- Pediatric Neurology Part I Christa Hutaff-Lee, ... Nicole Tartaglia, in Handbook of Clinical Neurology, 2013; Science Direct.
- Orphanet Journal of Rare Diseases 2007, 2:27 doi:10.1186/1750-1172-2-27 Ellis-Van Creveld syndrome.
- Mayo Clin Proc 67:549-552, 1992 Tibia Vara in a Patient With Bardet-Biedl Syndrome.

- American Family Physician September 15, 2003 / Volume 68, Number 6; Diagnostic Approach to Polyarticular Joint Pain.
- Can J Infect Dis Vol 6 No 3 May/June 1995 Poststreptococcal arthritis.
- University of Oklahoma Health Sciences Center; 2016- Streptococcus pyogenes : Basic Biology to Clinical Manifestations.
- Eur Cardiol. 2016 Aug; 11(1): 54–59 Uric Acid and Cardiovascular Disease: An Update.
- Harrison's Principle of Internal Medicine,19th Edition, Page 2136, Chapter 380.
- Circulation Volume 131, Issue 20, 19 May 2015, Pages 1806-1818 Revision of the Jones Criteria for the Diagnosis of Acute Rheumatic Fever in the Era of Doppler Echocardiography.

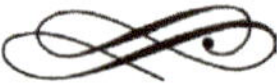

CHAPTER

2 Arterial Pulse

With the availability of sophisticated investigations these days, we usually subject the patients directly to these tests without thinking that clinical examination is equally important right at the first or grass root level when the patient meets the doctor in his OPD/casualty.

Arterial pulse, BP, JVP, Pedal edema, Basilar rales, etc are some of the most important cardiovascular findings that one should always look for and should not miss.

Arterial pulse is defined as an impulse that is generated due to abrupt arterial distension due to ejection of blood from the LV cavity to the aorta and then propelled further into the peripheral arterial tree. This impulse can travel at a speed > 20 times of that of the ejected blood bolus. Systolic BP is indicated by the peak of this arterial pulse.

The speed of pressure pulse transmission ⇒

Aorta: 3-5 m/s

Large arteries: 7-10 m/s

Small arteries: 15-35 m/s ,

where velocity is inversely proportional to the vascular compliance.

Pulse wave pattern

Carotid arterial pulse pattern is nearly the same as that of the central aortic pulse pressure because it is a large artery and is very close to the aortic valve.
Hence, the choices are ⇒

- Carotid artery: volume and contour
- Brachial artery: arterial wall condition
- Radial artery: rate and rhythm
- Femoral artery: pulsus paradoxus.

The arterial waveform pattern depends upon:

- Heart rate, stroke volume, arteriolar resistance, LVOT obstruction, peripheral vascular elasticity.

The aortic pulse wave has an initial sharp upstroke known as the PERCUSSION/INCIDENT wave which reflects the systolic ejection phase wherein the blood from the LV cavity is forced into the aorta. This wave occurs just after S1. Following this is a small crest called the ANACROTIC NOTCH reflecting propulsion of blood from aorta to the arteries of the periphery. Next to follow is the DICROTIC notch, which is a negative wave and indicates diastole and the lowermost point of which is called the INCISURA reflecting aortic valve closure and the positive wave indicates recoil from the aorta and aortic valve.

Normally, we can palpate only the systolic peak of the arterial pulse.

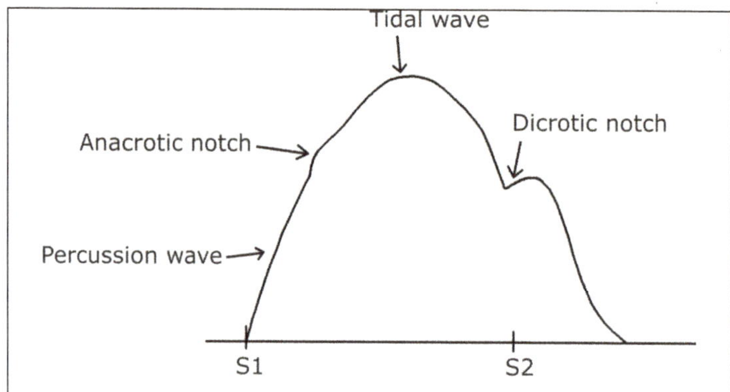

Fig. 2.1: Normal arterial pulse pattern.

The pulse pattern of the peripheral arteries are different from that of the aortic or carotid pulse, reflecting their muscular status and merging of the incident and the reflected waves.

Characteristics of the pulse wave of the peripheral arteries are:

- Steep upstroke
- High systolic peak
- Shorter time to systolic upstroke
- Increased pulse pressure
- Decreased MAP
- No anacrotic notch
- Smoother dicrotic notch

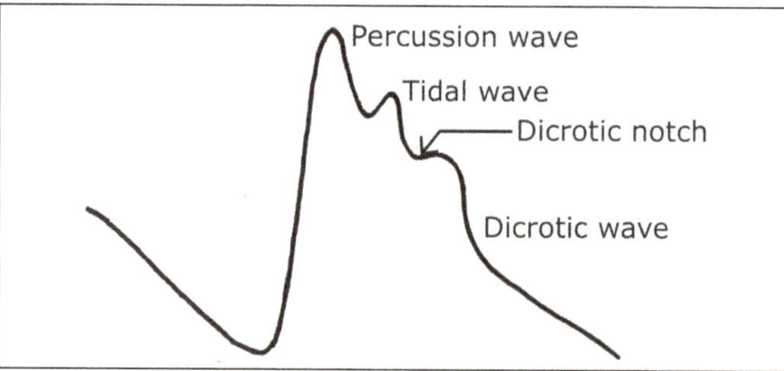

Fig. 2.2: Normal pulse wave in peripheral (brachial) artery.

However, when the pulse is released from the central aorta, it takes a small fraction of time to reach the peripheral sites and carotids as enumerated:

→ Carotids: 30 ms

→ Brachials: 60 ms

→ Femorals: 75 ms

→ Radials: 80 ms

Sites of Arterial Pulse Examination

Carotid artery: Patient lying on the bed with the trunk slightly elevated. Carotid artery felt with the thumb between the larynx and Sternocleidomastoid muscle anterior border. Examine one carotid at a time to avoid cerebral hypoperfusion. Also check for bruit by auscultation. The timing of the pulse can be improved by simultaneous auscultation of the heart beats.

A bruit is a vascular sound due to turbulence in blood flow due to stenosis.

The bruit character depends upon the pressure gradient developing due to the stenosis.

Vessel 50% stenosed → soft bruit in early systole

Vessel 60% stenosed → high pitched holosystolic bruit

Vessel 70-80% stenosed → systolic plus early diastolic bruit

Vessel completely stenosed → bruit disappears.

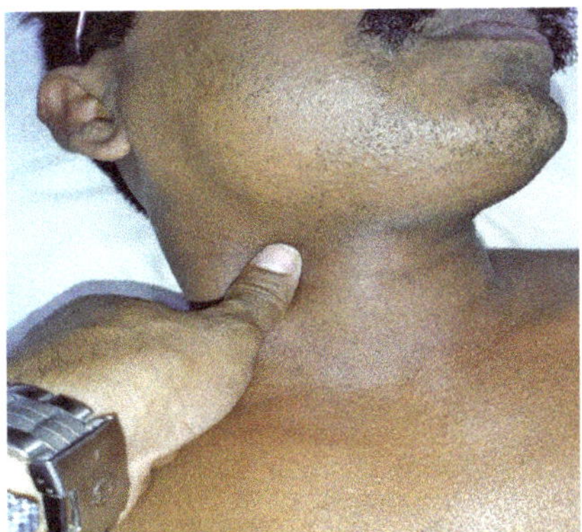

Fig. 2.3: Carotid pulse examination.

Radial artery: Best felt at the wrist, lateral to Flexor carpi radialis tendon and against the radius bone. It is palpated with the middle three fingers of the hand. The distal finger is used to empty the vessel, proximal finger palpates the pulse and middle finger judges the condition of the vessel wall. Radial pulse is used to check the rate and rhythm.

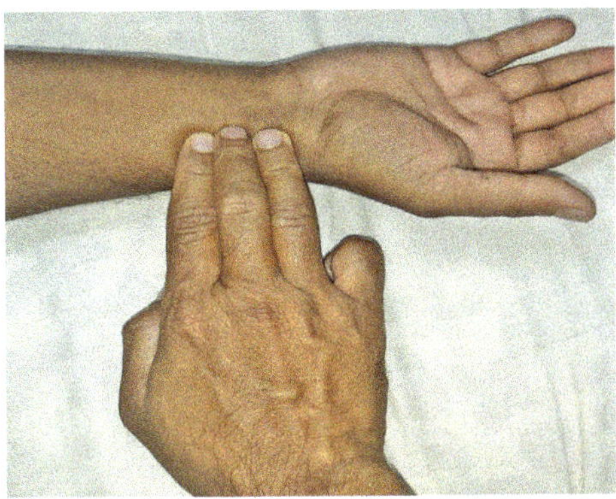

Fig. 2.4: Radial pulse examination.

Brachial artery: Best felt with the thumb (right thumb for right brachial artery) above the antecubital fossa and against the humerus bone, lateral to the tendon of the biceps muscle. It is a larger artery, hence can give ideas about the volume, and character of the pulse and also the condition of the vessel wall.

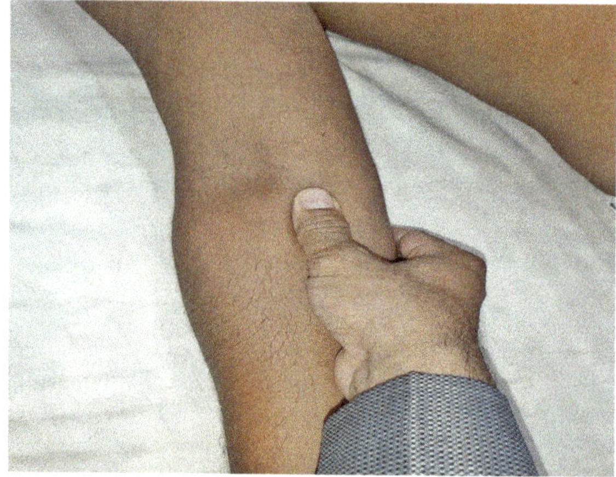

Fig. 2.5: Brachial pulse examination.

Femoral artery: Felt midway between the pubic ramus and the anterior superior iliac spine at the inguinal ligament level.

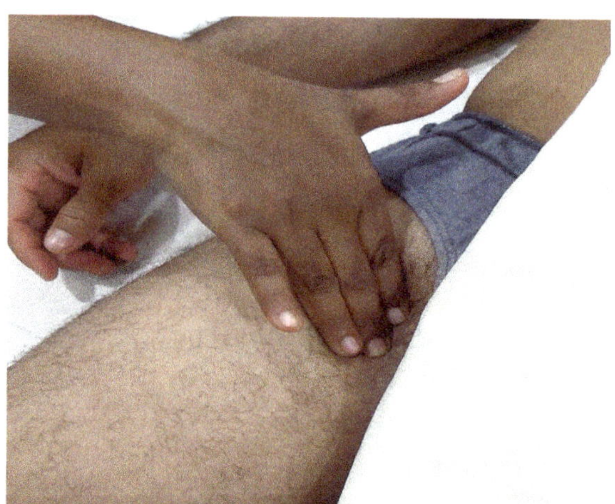

Fig. 2.6: Femoral artery examination.

Popliteal artery: Felt at the middle of the popliteal fossa with the patient lying supine with the knees slightly flexed (around 120^0).

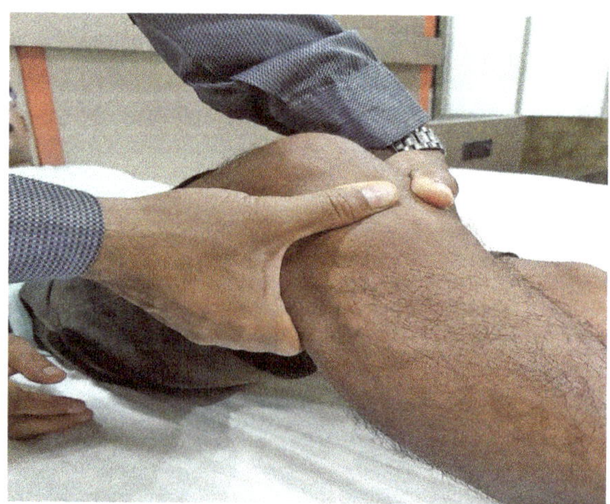

Fig. 2.7: Popliteal artery palpation.

Posterior tibial artery: Lies just posterior (around 1 cm) to the medial malleolus. The foot of the patient should be relaxed.

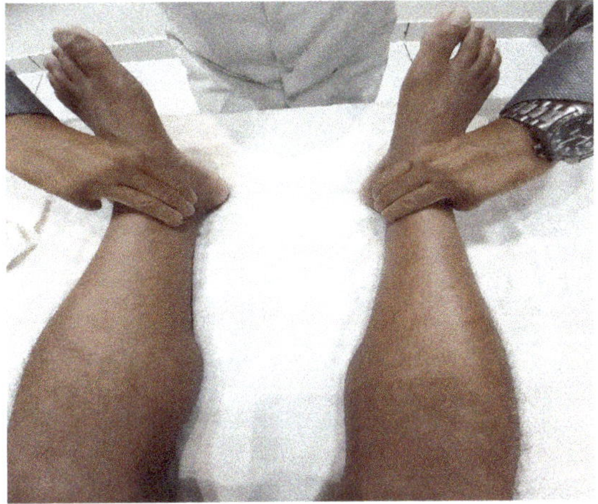

Fig. 2.8: Posterior tibial artery palpation.

Dorsalis pedis artery(DPA): Palpated with the middle three fingers of the hand (right hand for patients left DPA and vice versa) in the mid dorsum of the foot, just lateral to the extensor hallucis longus tendon.

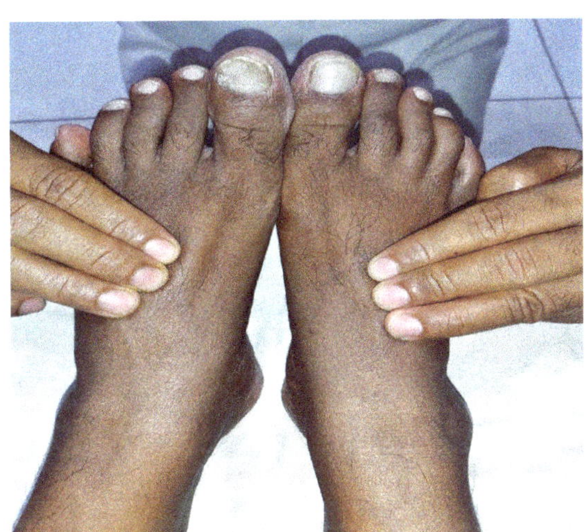

Fig. 2.9: Dorsalis pedis artery palpation.

Grading of the arterial pulse is done as follows →

→ Grade 0: Absent

→ Grade 1: Faintly detectable

→ Grade 2: Slightly diminished than normal

→ Grade 3: Normal

→ Grade 4: Bounding

When examining the pulse, variable pressure is applied to the artery with the finger pads to feel the waveforms (upstroke, systolic, diastolic etc) and this method is called "Trisection method".

The arterial pulse is checked for Rate, Rhythm, Character, Volume, Condition of the vessel wall, Bilateral symmetry, radiofemoral delay, etc.

RATE

The pulse should be counted for a whole 1 minute to get the pulse rate. However, one can also count the number of pulses for 15 seconds and then multiply it by 4 to get one minute pulse rate.

Normal pulse rate is 60-100 beats per minute.

Tachycardia is a pulse rate (sinus rate) > 100 beats per minute.

Bradycardia is a pulse rate (sinus rate) < 60 beats per minute.

Causes of tachycardia

Physiological → Infants, Exercise, Emotions.

Pathological → Anemia, fever, thyrotoxicosis, anterior wall MI, hypovolemia, drugs (atropine, nifedipine, beta2 agonists, thyroxine, catecholamines, caffeine, nicotine), tachyarrhythmias (SVT, atrial fibrillation, ventricular tachycardia, etc).

Causes of bradycardia

Physiological→ Sleep, athletes.

Pathological→ Hypothermia, myxedema, obstructive jaundice, inferior wall MI, increased ICT, drugs (beta blockers, verapamil, propafenone, lithium, digoxin), bradyarrhythmias (heart blocks).

Sinus arrhythmia

→ Variation of normal rhythm

→ It is an ECG finding

→ Respiratory variation of P-P interval of > 0.12 seconds (pulse rate↑ with inspiration and ↓ with expiration, called phasic sinus arrhythmia)

→ It occurs due to intermittent vagal stimulation and changes in cardiac pressure during respiration

→ Its presence is indicative of a good cardiac health and absence is suggestive of heart failure or other cardiac illnesses like a large ASD.

Apex pulse deficit

→ Counting the difference between the radial pulse rate and the actual heart rate by auscultation is a very important test to differentiate between Atrial fibrillation and Ventricular premature beats.

→ It occurs due to a reduction of preload in tachyarrhythmias which leads to a reduced LVEF that causes an inadequate opening of the aortic valve that fails to produce an appreciable radial pulse despite a heart beat.

→ This test can be performed either by two people, one calculating the radial pulse and the other counting the heart beats by auscultation or can be done by a single person who palpates the radial pulse with one hand and checks the heartbeat with a stethoscope and directly counts the number of heart beats that do not reach the radial artery over 1 minute duration.

→ An apex pulse deficit (APD) > 6 beats per minute is suggestive of atrial fibrillation and an APD < 6 beats per minute suggest premature ventricular contraction.

RHYTHM

Normal rhythm of the pulse is regular or sinus rhythm, indicating that the impulse is generated through the SA node.

It is assessed through the radial artery.

If irregular, we should check whether it is IRREGULARLY IRREGULAR OR REGULARLY IRREGULAR.

Irregularly irregular rhythm: atrial fibrillation, multiple ventricular ectopics, atrial tachyarrhythmias with varying AV blocks.

Regularly irregular rhythm: sinus arrhythmia, VPCs (bigeminy, trigemini), 1^0 and 2^0 AV blocks.

CHARACTER

Character of the pulse is assessed with the help of the carotid pulse.

Some of the abnormal characters are discussed below.

Pulsus parvus et tardus

→ This type of pulse is seen in severe valvular aortic stenosis.

→ This pulse has a slow rising (parvus) nature with a delayed systolic peak (tardus) and upstroke with a low volume.

→ The slow rising nature is due to fixed obstruction at the LVOT level, and indicates a pressure gradient of minimum 70 mmHg at the aortic valve level.

→ This can be best felt if one auscultates the heart and simultaneously palpates the carotid pulse.

→ The low volume of the pulse is due to increased systemic vascular resistance.

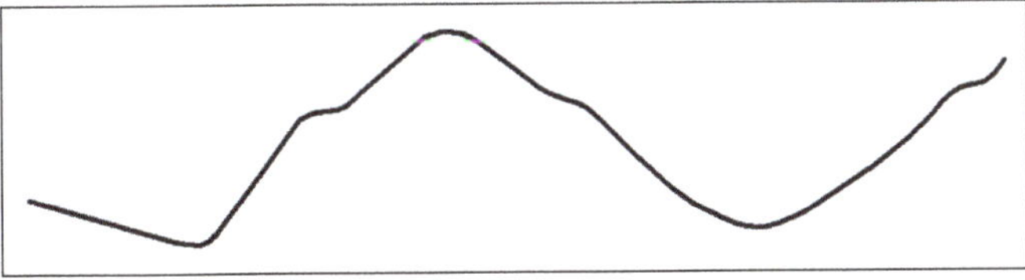

Fig. 2.10: Pulsus parvus et tardus in Aortic stenosis.

Water hammer pulse (Collapsing/Corrigan) pulse:

→ First described by Dr. D.J. Corrigan

→ Dr. Thomas Watson compared this pulse to the Water-hammer toy which has a tube half filled with water and half vacuum and that produces a sound which resembles a hammer blow.

→ This pulse is a hyper bounding pulse with a rapid upstroke and a rapid downstroke without a dicrotic notch.

→ Aortic regurgitation: MC condition causing water hammer pulse.

→ The rapid upstroke is due to an ↑ stroke volume because in AR there is an increase in the End-diastolic volume due to some blood going back to the LV cavity during diastole due to incompetent aortic valves.

→ The rapid downstroke is due to the aortic "run-off" of blood in the LV during diastole, and also due to rapid emptying of the arterial system due to reduced systemic vascular resistance.

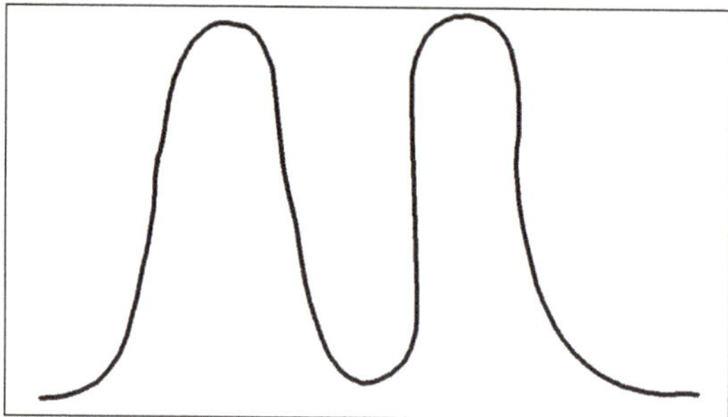

Fig. 2.11: Water hammer pulse.

→ To examine the water hammer pulse, the patient's wrist is held in a wrapping manner by the examiner's hand and radial pulsations felt (patient in supine and slightly inclined position). The patient's hand is then lifted above the head which makes the artery more aligned to the aorta and makes the water hammer pulse to be felt clearly as a tapping impulse due to rapid emptying of blood from the upper limb during diastole due to gravity.

→ Causes of water hammer pulse: Exercise, fever, pregnancy, anemia, beri beri, thyrotoxicosis, AV fistula, AR, MR, PDA, truncus arteriosus, complete heart block, sinus of Valsalva rupture, etc.

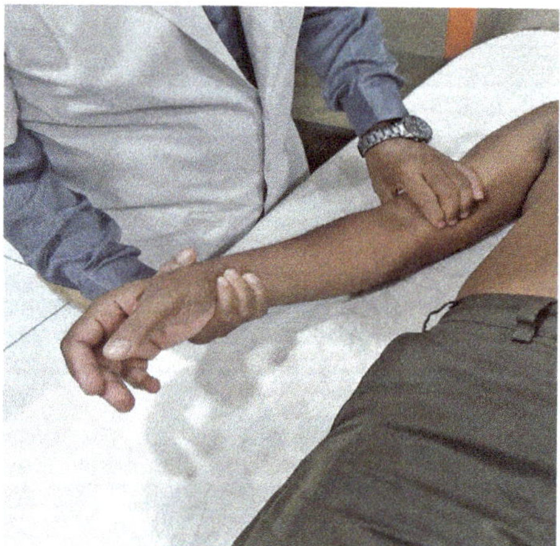

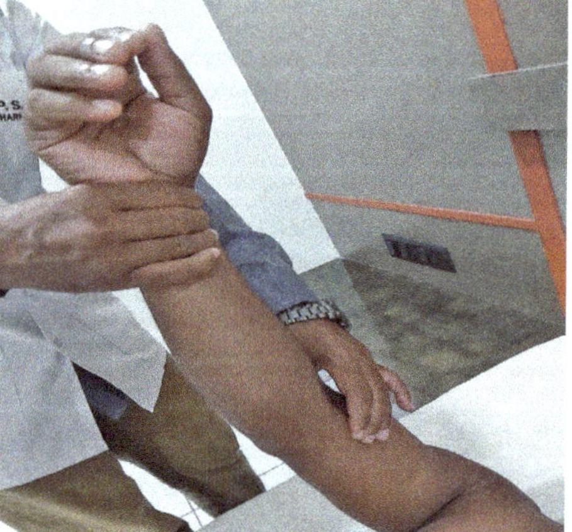

Fig. 2.12: Technique of detecting the WATER HAMMER pulse.

Anacrotic pulse

→ Slow rising (pulsus tardus), twice beating pulse (anacrotic and tidal waves), both of which are felt in systole.

→ Seen in aortic stenosis.

Pulsus Bisferiens

→ Single pulse wave but with two peaks (percussion wave and tidal wave), both of which are in systole.

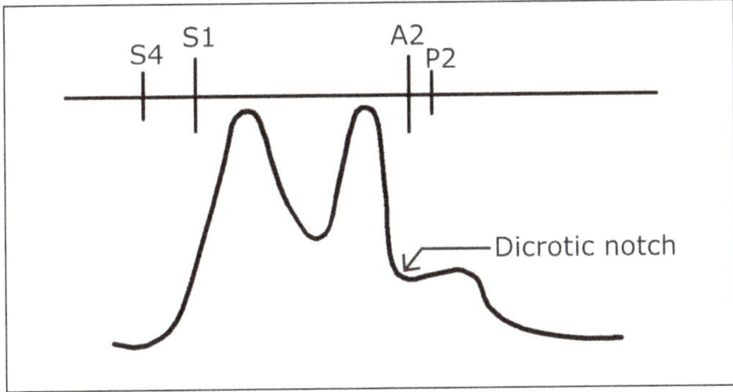

Fig. 2.13

→ Causes: AR with AS, hypertrophic obstructive cardiomyopathy (HOCM), severe AR, aortic dissection (unilateral bisferiens).

→ Usually the percussion wave is felt and not the tidal wave which is due to aortic recoil and reflection from the periphery. But any condition that exaggerates the percussion wave would exaggerate the tidal wave as well.

→ In combined AR plus AS, the stenotic lesion leads to the formation of a high velocity jet due pressure gradients. But by the Bernoulli phenomenon, there is a fall in pressure on the lateral part of this jet leading to the formation of a dip in the pulse with a secondary tidal wave (slow rising and collapsing pulses).

→ In HOCM, the LVOT obstruction due to systolic anterior motion and ventricular hypertrophy occurs in mid- or late systole. In the earlier part of LV ejection is normal and rapid leading to the rapid upstroke. In the late systole due to the sudden dynamic obstruction, there is a dip in the pressure pulse followed by a slowly rising pulse. Hence, the pulse in HOCM has components of both, AR (initial steep upstroke) and AS (slowly rising pulse).

→ It is better felt over the brachial; or the radial arteries because carotid shudder may mask the features over the carotid artery. It is felt by applying slow and graduated pressure over the artery to be able to feel the two separate waves. Alternatively, we can completely obliterate the pulse and then slowly release the pressure until a point where we feel the two waves.

Dicrotic pulse

→ Dicrotic wave - reflection from periphery.

→ Seen commonly in states of low cardiac output with ↓ peripheral resistance like tamponade, myocarditis etc.

→ It is a single pulse wave with two peaks, one in systole and the other one in diastole.

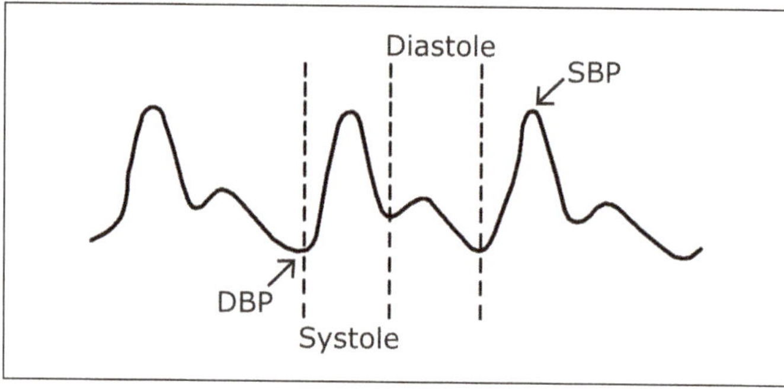

Fig. 2.14

→ The second wave of dicrotic pulse occurs after the second heart sound, a point that helps differentiate it from bisferiens pulse.

→ Better felt in the radial artery and on inspiration.

→ Dicrotic pulse does not occur if the systolic BP is > 130 mmHg.

→ Causes: Enteric fever, LVF, dilated cardiomyopathy, dehydration, myocarditis, cardiac tamponade.

Pulsus bigeminus:

→ Alternate strong and weak beats

→ Occur irregularly (unlike pulsus alternans)

→ The weaker beat remains close to the previous normal beat and is followed by a lengthy pause.

→ The stronger beat occurs after the long pause and is due to increased LV end diastolic volume due to post extrasystolic potentiation (due to ↑ diastolic filling time due to the long pause).

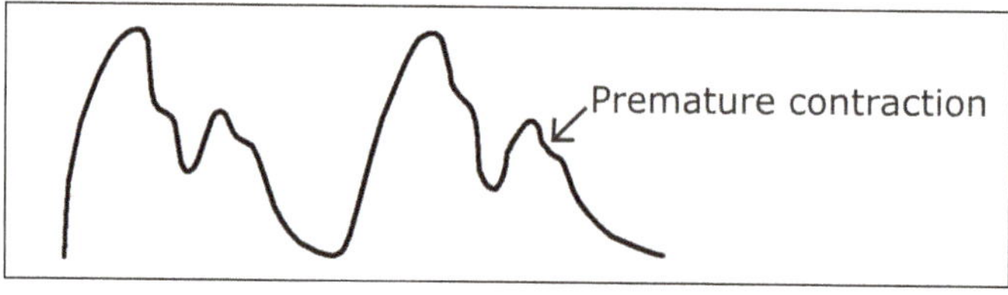

Fig. 2.15

→ However, in conditions like HOCM, the post extrasystolic potentiation may actually increase the obstruction to LVOT leading to a fall in pulse volume.

This failure of rise of the beat by ≥ 10 mmHg or an actual fall in pulse is popularly known as **BROCKENBROUGH-BRAUNWALD SIGN** (rise in LV systolic pressure with a paradoxical fall in pulse pressure).

This can also be seen in LV dysfunction and constrictive pericarditis.

Pulsus alternans

→ Discovered by Traube.

→ Regular rhythm pulse with alternate strong and weak beats.

→ Can be detected by a sphygmomanometer by detecting the alternation of the Korotkoff sound intensity.

→ Occurs due to severe ventricular depression and indicates a lesser number of contractile elements involved in cardiac contractions.

→ MC condition causing pulsus alternans is aortic stenosis with cardiac failure

→ Alternans total: LV systolic pressure < aortic diastolic pressure ⇒ aortic valve fails to open.

→ Alternans concordant: Both sides of the heart involved (R and L ventricles).

→ Alternans discordant: When only one side of the heart is involved (either R or L ventricle).

→ Factors exaggerating Pulsus alternans: AR, Hypertension, head tilting or giving nitroglycerine (it ↓ venous return).

→ Electrical alternans (beat to beat variation of QRS complex amplitude) seen in massive pericardial effusion has got nothing to do with pulsus alternans.

→ Pulsus alternans can be detected by palpating the peripheral pulses if the aortic pressure alternates by > 20 mmHg.

→ Patient should hold the breath in mid expiration during the examination.

→ Causes: Severe AS with LVF, severe AR with LVF, DCM, PS, myocarditis, acute pulmonary embolism, etc.

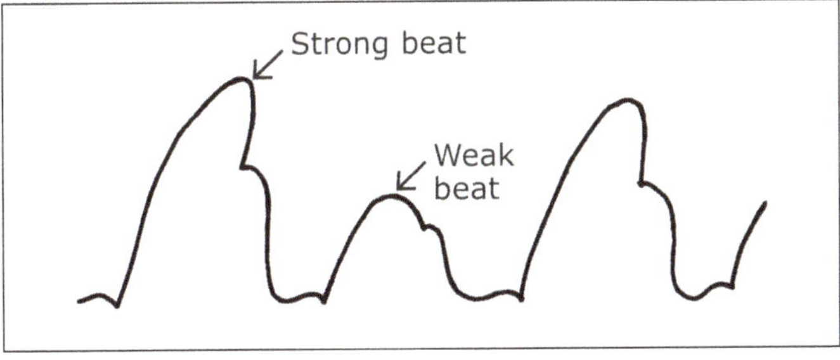

Fig. 2.16: Pulsus alternans.

Pulsus paradoxus

→ Discovered by Adolf Kussmaul in 1873.

→ Defined as an inspiratory fall of SBP > 10 mmHg.

→ Normally, the SBP doesn't fall > 8 mmHg during inspiration.

→ Normal changes in heart during respiration:

- During inspiration, the right atrial pressure decreases due to a decrease in the intrathoracic pressure (ITP) which causes an increased blood flow from the vena cavae to the right atrium.
- This ↑ right atrial filling increases the RV end diastolic volume (RVEDV) which leads to a rise in the intrapericardial pressure leading to increased left atrial pressure and decreased left atrial filling. Also, the ↑ RVEDV during inspiration causes the septum to shift to the left leading to ↓ LV compliance(Parallel biventricular interdependence).
- The RV stroke volume takes some time to pass through the lungs to go to the LV known as the Pulmonary transit time (PTT). Now because the PTT is slightly long (5-10 seconds), the stroke volume which is increased on the right side during inspiration can be increased on the left side only during expiration (because respiration is a continuous and cyclic process obviously)(Series biventricular interdependence).
- Thus the decrease in the Left atrial filling during inspiration can be attributed to: (1) series biventricular interdependence (interaction), (2) Parallel ventricular interdependence, and (3) ↓ LV diastolic time due to increased heart rate during inspiration.
- Hence, there is a normal fall of SBP during inspiration (not > 8 mmHg) (Hence, jokingly I feel that pulsus paradoxus can also be called as pulsus aggravatus).

→ Causes of pulsus paradoxus: Cardiac tamponade(MC), severe asthma, constrictive pericarditis, severe COPD, morbid obesity, voluntary deep inspiration(student paradoxus), pregnancy, etc.

→ Mechanism of pulsus paradoxus in cardiac tamponade: In cardiac tamponade, the inspiratory ↑ in RVEDV cannot be accommodated as in normal patients. Hence, the RV distension causes an exaggerated deviation of the septum towards the left leading to ↓ LV end diastolic volume and hence a ↓ stroke volume during inspiration.The reverse of this phenomenon takes place in expiration.

→ Mechanism of pulsus paradoxus in asthma or COPD: Varying swings in ITP and deep respiratory movements.

→ Mechanism of pulsus paradoxus in obesity: marked alterations of ITP and increased work of breathing.

→ Clinical determination of Pulsus paradoxus:

- Femoral arteries are best suited.

- Sphygmomanometer is used.
- First determine the systolic blood pressure of the patient.
- Then inflate the arm cuff to a pressure just above this systolic pressure. The pressure is then reduced very slowly (≈ 2 mmHg/beat) to find the pressure at which the first Korotkoff sounds are first heard, usually only in expiration. The pressure is further lowered to get a pressure at which the sounds are audible both in expiration and inspiration. Pulsus paradoxus is detected if the pressure difference reading between the former and the latter is > 10 mmHg.
- Significant pulsus paradoxus ⇒ >15 mmHg fall of pressure.
- Pulsus paradoxus may be absent in any lesion that prevents the reduced LV filling during inspiration, e.g.; AR which increases the amount of blood in LV or any shunt lesion (ASD, VSD) which equalizes the biventricular pressures.
- **Reversed pulsus paradoxus** is when there is an expiratory fall of SBP and is seen in positive pressure ventilation (ITP higher during inspiration), HOCM, and Isorhythmic ventricular rhythm.

VOLUME OF THE PULSE

The palpating finger feels for the pulse amplitude.
Volume depends on the pulse pressure.

Pulsus magnus

→ High volume pulse due to ↑ stroke volume.

→ Seen in aortic regurgitation.

Hyperkinetic pulse

→ Also called bounding pulse.

→ Large amplitude pulse.

→ Seen in hyperdynamic circulatory states, MR, VSD, etc.

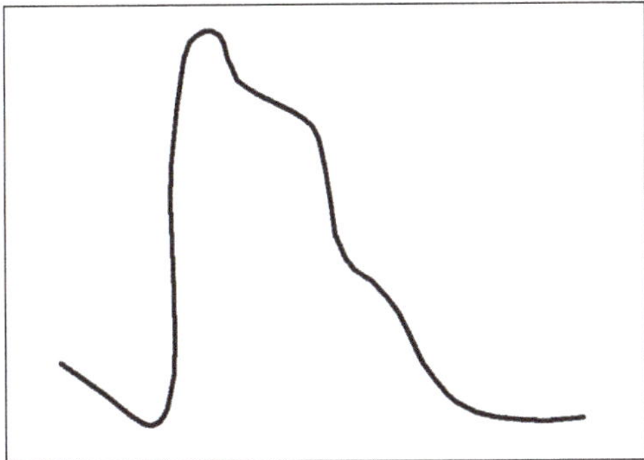

Fig. 2.17: Hyperkinetic pulse.

Hypokinetic pulse

→ Weak pulse with narrow pulse pressure.

→ Seen in shock, heart failure, MS, AS.

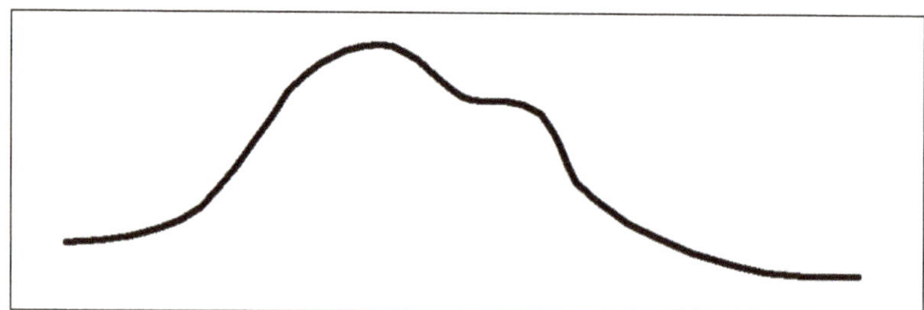

Fig. 2.18: Hypokinetic pulse.

BILATERAL SYMMETRY

One should check all the pulses bilaterally.

Asymmetrical pulses are commonly seen in:

→ Takayasu arteritis

→ Cervical rib (thoracic outlet syndrome)

→ Long standing atherosclerosis

→ Micro Embolisms

→ Aortic dissection

→ Subclavian steal syndrome

CONDITION OF THE VESSEL WALL

Apply pressure on the artery with the finger and try to roll it to feel the consistency.

Usually in young people we cannot feel the artery whereas in the older population the artery may feel like a thick cord due to atherosclerosis.

RADIOFEMORAL DELAY

Palpate the radial and femoral pulses simultaneously.

A delay in femoral pulse arrival is indicative of:

→ Coarctation of aorta: decreased rate of rise of the amplitude

→ Peripheral artery disease involving aortic bifurcation, common iliac artery, external iliac artery, etc.

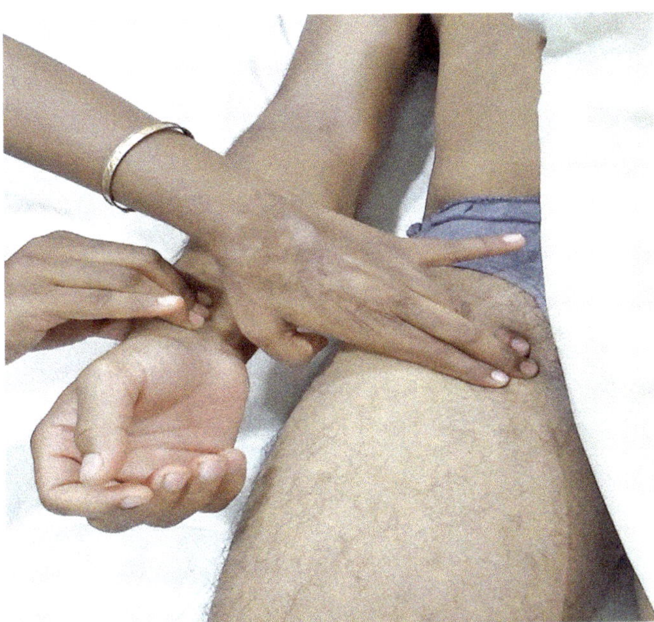

Fig. 2.19: Checking for radio-femoral delay.

References

- APIINDIA Chapter 195 Back to Bedside Basics - Pulse, Blood Pressure and Jugular Venous Pulse.
- Clinical Methods: The history, physical, and Laboratory Examinations. 3rd edition Chapter 20 The Carotid Pulse.
- Clinical Methods: The history, physical, and Laboratory Examinations. 3rd edition Chapter 30 Examination of the Extremities : Pulses, Bruits, and Phlebitis.
- Clinical Methods: The history, physical, and Laboratory Examinations. 3rd edition Chapter 18 Bruits and Hums of the Head and Neck.
- Macleod's Clinical examination 12th edition Chapter 6 The cardiovascular system.
- Guyton and Hall Textbook of Medical Physiology, 12th Ed CHAPTER 15 Vascular Distensibility and Functions of the Arterial and Venous Systems.
- Braunwald's Heart Disease 8th edition Chapter 11 The History and Physical Examination: An evidence-based approach.
- J Cardiol. 1988 Mar;18(1):197-205 Mechanism of production of pulse deficit in atrial fibrillation: assessment by blood flow dynamics.
- StatPearls [Internet] Sinus Arrhythmia.
- Treasure Island (FL): StatPearls Publishing; 2020 Jan-. Water Hammer Pulse.
- Clinical methods in Cardiology by B Soma Raju.
- Eur Respir J 2013; 42: 1696–1705 | DOI: 10.1183/09031936.00138912 Pulsus paradoxus.
- METHODIST DEBAKEY CARDIOVASC J | 14 (4) 2018 Reversed Pulsus Paradoxus in Right Ventricular Failure.

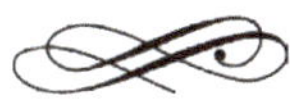

CHAPTER

3 Blood Pressure

Arterial pressure or blood pressure (BP) is the pressure in the arteries which is exerted by the blood.

It depends on the cardiac output (CO) and the total peripheral resistance.

CO= Stroke volume (SV) x Heart rate (HR)

↑SV increases SBP

↑HR increases DBP

Expressed as mmHG or kPa.

1 mmHg = 0.13332 kPa

There are several components of the blood pressure:

Systolic BP (SBP)

→ Due to cardiac contraction.

→ Normally < 120 mmHg.

→ It depends on CO, arterial elasticity, blood viscosity.

Diastolic BP (DBP)

→ Reflects the cardiac relaxation.

→ Normally < 80 mmHg.

→ It depends on the blood velocity and the total peripheral resistance.

Pulse pressure (PP)

→ SBP minus DBP

→ Normally 40 mmHg

→ It is a determinant for pulse volume and arterial stiffness.

Mean blood pressure (MBP)

→ MBP = DBP+1/3PP

→ It determines the perfusion pressure for every organ in the body

→ Normally it is around 70 to 100 mmHg.

- → MAP < 60 mmHG can lead to tissue hypoperfusion leading to renal failure, neural abnormalities, shock, etc.

MEASUREMENT OF BLOOD PRESSURE

Direct method

Involves arterial catheterization which seems impractical in the era when BP is measured non-invasively.

It is invasive and not possible for rapid execution.

Sometimes require brief sedation as well.

Indirect method

Includes sphygmomanometer method, oscillometric method, ultrasound doppler, home BP monitoring, ambulatory BP monitoring.

Sphygmomanometer Method (Mercury Sphygmomanometer)

- → The brachial artery is the standard location.
- → As we go to the more peripheral arteries, SBP increases and DBP decreases.
- → Auscultatory method with mercury sphygmomanometer - 'gold standard' for office blood pressure measurement(office BP means the healthcare visit BP taken to diagnose hypertension in a patient).
- → The BP measurement is usually done in the sitting posture because most of the research and literature available have studied the patients in sitting position only.

  The sphygmomanometer should be at the same level as that of the heart(right atrium).
- → The cuff size is very important. A very small and tight cuff would give an abnormally high BP and a large and loose cuff would give a falsely low BP.
- → Before starting the measurement, one should palpate the brachial artery first and then place the cuff in such a way that the centre of the bladder lies above the brachial artery. However, the arm of the patient should be bare and the arm sleeves of the shirt should not be rolled up as they can exert a tourniquet effect. Also, the lower edge of the cuff should be at least 2-3 cm above the antecubital fossa so that a Stethoscope can be placed on it.
- → Normal bladder cuff length: 75-100% of the arm circumference.
- → Normal bladder cuff width: 37-50% of the arm circumference.
- → The auscultatory sphygmomanometer method is always preceded by the palpatory method wherein the cuff is inflated upto a level where the brachial artery obstruction leads to disappearance of the radial artery pulse by palpation. The cuff is then deflated slowly and the pressure reading where the radial pulse just reappears is noted - which is the SBP.

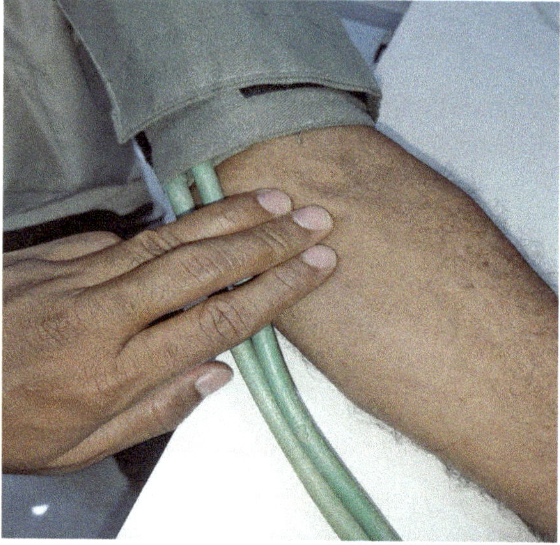

Fig. 3.1: The palpatory method of BP measurement.

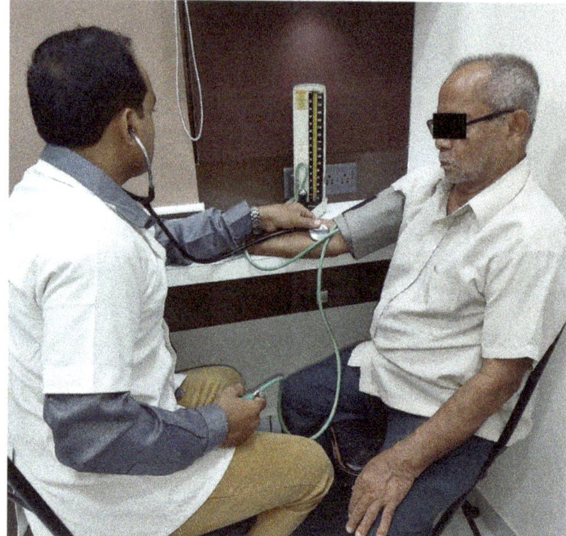

Fig. 3.2: The auscultatory method of BP measurement.

→ For the auscultatory method, the cuff is inflated to a pressure 30 mmHg above the SBP obtained by the palpatory method. The cuff is then deflated slowly at the rate of 2-3 mmHg to listen for the Korotkoff sounds over the brachial artery with the help of a Stethoscope. These sounds are produced due to the re-establishment of blood flow during deflation of the cuff.

→ If the cuff is deflated faster than 3 mmHg, one may miss the proper level of occurrence of the Korotkoff sound.

→ If the cuff is deflated too slowly, it would lead to slightly higher diastolic pressure.

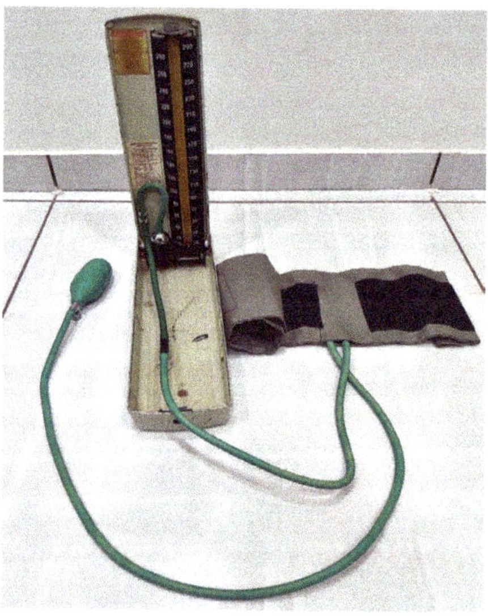

Fig. 3.3: Mercury Sphygmomanometer.

- The various phases of occurrence of Korotkoff sounds are:
  - Phase I - first appearance of a tapping sound during deflating the cuff and corresponds to the SBP.
  - Phase II - Tapping sound changing to a soft murmur. The silent auscultatory gap occurs if one misses this phase II.
  - Phase III - Augmented murmur
  - Phase IV - Muffling of the sound suddenly
  - Phase V - Disappearance of all the sounds and corresponds to the DBP.

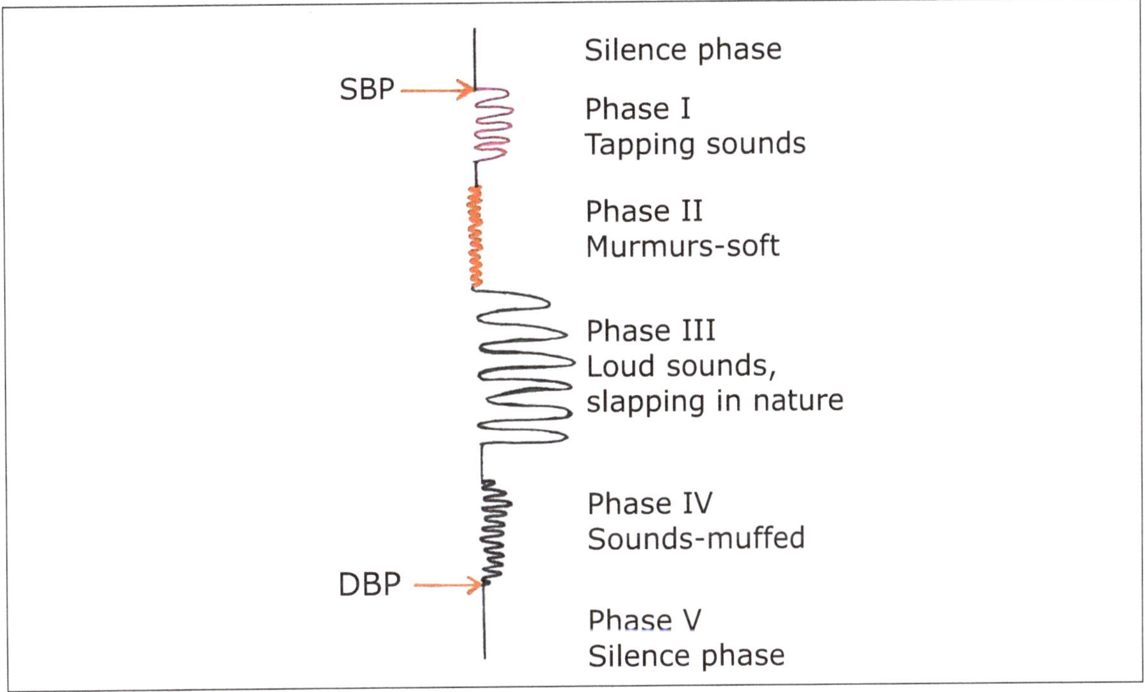

Fig. 3.4: Korotkoff sounds.

Auscultatory gap

- It is a sudden disappearance and the reappearance of the Korotkoff sounds between systolic and diastolic pressures during deflation of the cuff.
- It may lead to falsely high DBP or low SBP.
- The sound reappears well above the DBP and the radial pulse is felt during the silent phase.
- Usually occurs between phases I and II.
- May occur due to phasic alterations of arterial pressure or weak Korotkoff sounds.

→ The only way to avoid this gap is to confirm the SBP by palpatory method first and then obtaining the proper inflation pressure while doing the auscultatory method.

→ May be associated with target organ damage.

→ For example, the real SBP is 180 mmHg and the sound fades at 176 mmHg and again reappears at 160 mmHg and disappears at 106 mmHg.

If proper inflation pressure is not achieved, the doctor would record the BP as 160/106 mmHg instead of 180/106 mmHg. However, even if you achieve the proper inflation pressure above 200 mmHg (for example) and do not deflate properly, then too you will wrongly record the pressure as 180/176 mmHg. Hence, make it a habit to deflate the cuff uptil zero mark.

Some recommendations about the recording of BP

(1) ≥ 2 BP readings should be taken at the clinic visit, each separated by at least 2 minutes. For the diagnosis of hypertension, a minimum of 3 recordings are required at least 1 week apart.

(2) BP should be taken in both the arms in the initial visits and the arm with the higher BP should be considered at subsequent follow up visits. Usually the BP difference between both the arms should be <10 mmHg.

Conditions with SBP difference >10 mmHg between the two arms includes: Coarctation of aorta, subclavian steal syndrome, supravalvular aortic stenosis, thoracic outlet syndrome, arterial thrombosis etc.

(3) The patient should sit comfortably with his back supported and the feet flat on the ground. The patient should relax for 3-5 minutes without talking before the first BP recording is done. (If the back is not supported, the BP can be falsely high).

(4) No caffeine, exercise or smoking, minimum 30 minutes before measurement.

(5) Patient should empty his/her bladder.

(6) Record the SBP and DBP in even values only.

(7) Always make a note of the time if the patient has taken any BP treatment and medication.

(8) Always make it a habit to inform the BP readings to the patient, both verbally and in writing.

(9) The right atrium corresponds to the midpoint of the sternum or the fourth intercostal space in seated position.

(10) Supine subjects may have falsely raised BP compared to seated subjects (SBP - 3 to 10 mmHg, DBP - 1 to 5 mmHg).

(11) A patient sitting with crossed legs can have falsely raised BP.

Recoding BP in the Lower limbs

→ The patient is placed in a prone position.

→ The popliteal artery is palpated and the cuff is wrapped with the artery in the centre of the bladder (preferably use an 8 inch cuff).

→ The bottom edge of the cuff should be at least 1 inch above the bend of the knee for auscultation.

→ Similarly we can wrap the cuff on the calf and auscultate the posterior tibial artery or the dorsalis pedis artery.

→ Normally, the difference of SBP between the lower limb and the upper limb is < 20 mmHg.

A difference > 20 mmHg is seen in severe aortic regurgitation and is called Hill's sign.

→ Other causes of Hill's sign are: Coarctation of aorta, dissection of aorta, subclavian steal syndrome etc.

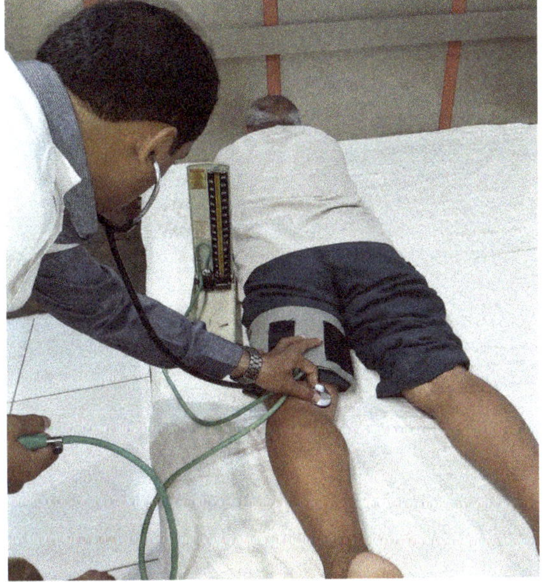

Fig. 3.5: BP recording in lower limb.

BP recording in Atrial fibrillation (AF)

The BP varies from beat to beat in AF. Hence, a mean of at least 3 recordings from each limb is taken and reported.

BP recording in Aortic regurgitation (AR)

It is well known that in severe AR, there is ↑LVEDV and diastolic 'run off' which gives rise to a high SBP and very low DBP. Sometimes the Korotkoff sounds don't disappear and are audible till the mercury column touches zero. But DBP cannot be zero obviously. Hence, in such cases the Phase IV Korotkoff sound is taken as the DBP (muffling of the sound). Hence, if the SBP is 180 mmHg (suppose) and the Phase IV sound occurs at 30 mmHg (suppose), then the BP is reported as 180/30-0 mmHg indicating that the Korotkoff sound was audible till zero reading.

Aneroid Sphygmomanometer

- → It is a non-automated, auscultatory, mercury free sphygmomanometer.
- → Consists of an aneroid gauge with a metal bellows with a watch-like movement due to pressure cuff and a pivoted pointer on a calibration dial.
- → These are subject to frequent errors.
- → Frequent calibration is needed for these devices (6 monthly for wall mounted and every 2 to 4 weeks for the handheld one).

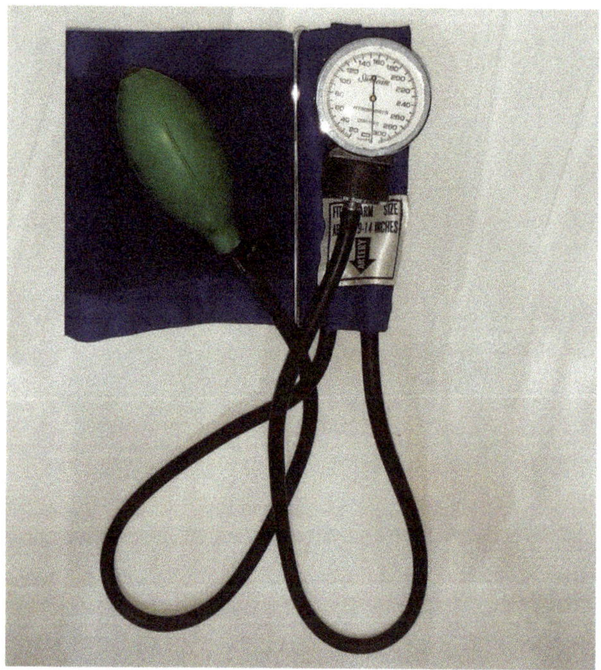

Fig. 3.6: Aneroid Sphygmomanometer.

Hybrid sphygmomanometer

- → Auscultatory, non-automated, mercury free device.
- → There is a free moving liquid crystal column that moves like a mercury column only.
- → However, the observer must auscultate for the Korotkoff sounds and record the BP.
- → These devices are quite reliable.

Oscillometric devices

→ Detects the amplitude of oscillations in the upper part of the lateral arm.

→ Commonly used for home, clinic, ambulatory settings, hence do not need special training to use.

→ MAP is detected very accurately in addition to SBP and DBP.

→ Each device has their own proprietary algorithm which is manufacturer specific. Hence, the devices are not interchangeable.

→ Electronic oscillometric sphygmomanometer for home use usually measures one BP recording at a time. But oscillometric sphygmomanometers designed for hospitals can record multiple readings at a time, although quite expensive.

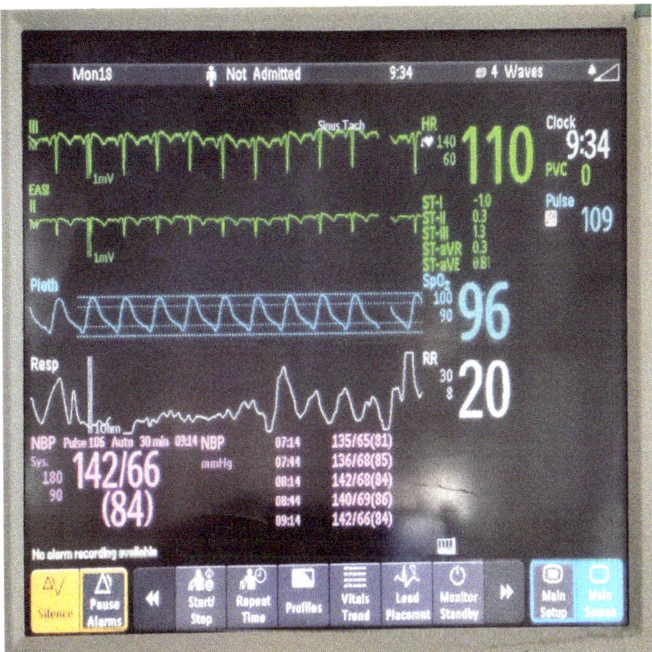

Fig. 3.7

Ultrasonography techniques

→ Non invasive technique.

→ The ultrasound transducer placed over the surface of the artery detects the absolute BP waveforms.

→ Used for patients with weaker Korotkoff sounds and those with difficult arterial access like the patients of AV fistula on maintenance dialysis.

→ Very accurate for measuring SBP.

Tonometry

→ Non invasive method

→ Gives good representation of the aortic pressure waveforms.

→ A handheld tonometer is held on the radial artery with mild pressure.

→ The machine sensor then records the radial artery pressures digitally.

→ The central pressure indices are then calculated using Fourier analysis.

→ SBP and DBP are obtained from the waveform shapes.

→ However, the devices are operator dependent, and need proper training and calibration.

Wrist monitors

→ These are small devices and can be used in obese people.

→ The only major issue is that there could be error due to variable wrist positions relative to the heart.

→ This can be corrected if the wrist is at the level of the heart, but then it is not possible to guess when the device is going to review the BP.

→ These devices need further evaluation.

Finger monitors

→ Usually not accurate and better avoided.

Flush technique

→ Used for the detection of coarctation of aorta in infants.

→ The limb is elevated and elastic bandage is wrapped from the fingertips or toes and progressed proximally towards the wrist or ankle so that blood in the skin capillaries and veins is eliminated and the limb blanches. A sphygmomanometer cuff (of pediatric

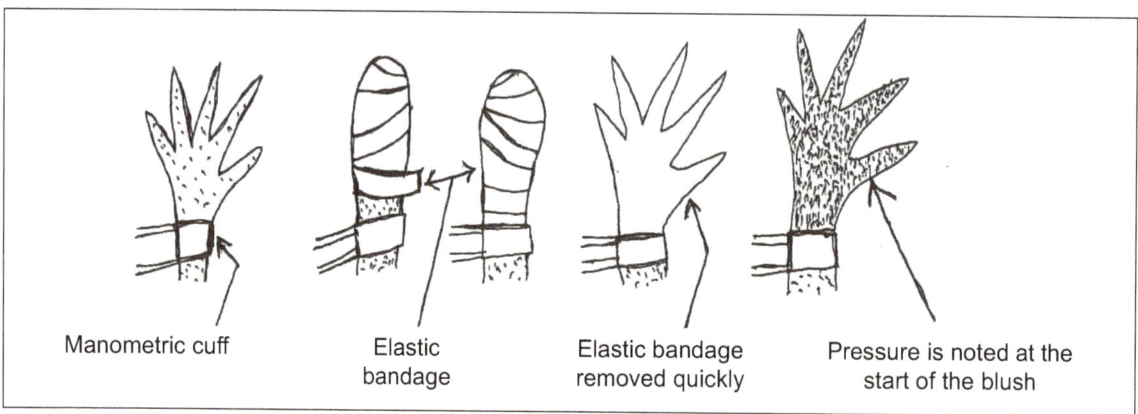

Fig. 3.8: The Flush Technique.

size) is then applied to the wrist or the ankle and inflated 30 mmHg above the SBP. The bandage is then removed keeping the cuff in place so that the limb remains blanched. The cuff is then deflated by 2-3 mmHg per second and attention is paid to the pressure at which the skin first starts blushing. This pressure is considered as the MAP.

Ambulatory BP monitoring (ABPM)

- Non invasive, automated procedure.
- Oscillometric devices are used that record the BP over a 24 hour period usually in patients > 40 years of age.
- ABPM associated BP is a better indicator of target organ damage and bad CVS outcome.
- Usually the non dominant arm is selected so that the daily activities do not interfere with the machine.
- The patient should be explained about the procedure, and the fact that the ABPM process may disrupt his sleep. Patient should avoid taking a shower or swimming, note his meal and sleep time, and also the timing of taking any antihypertensive medication, if any.
- The patient should also note the time of any adverse event(s) like vertigo, palpitation, breathlessness, headache, etc.
- The machine usually records the BP every 15-30 minutes in the whole 24 hour period.
- The international recommendation for the minimum number of readings that the machine should take are ≥ 20 day time readings and ≥ 7 night time readings.
- Indications of ABPM:
  - White coat/masked hypertension
  - Monitoring antihypertensive treatment efficacy
  - Nocturnal hypertension
  - Postural hypotension
  - Postprandial hypotension
  - Drug induced hypotension
  - Hypotension due to autonomic dysfunction

Home BP monitoring

- It minimizes the chances of White coat hypertension.
- Multiple readings are possible over a prolonged period.
- Helps in predicting target organ damage and cardiovascular prognosis.
- Automated oscillometric devices with memory chips are good for home BP recordings.

Nocturnal hypertension

→ Raised BP during sleep

→ Detected by ABPM

→ More common among patients of diabetes mellitus and chronic kidney disease

→ Associated with ↑ risk of cardiovascular events.

Diurnal variation of BP

→ Normally there is a 10-20 mmHg dip in the BP during sleep with a rise in the morning after waking up.

→ The BP is usually highest after 6 am until noon.

→ The nocturnal dipping of BP is lost in Malignant hypertension, chronic kidney disease, autonomic neuropathy, etc.

→ This night time rise of BP has been found to be associated with ↑ cardiovascular disease risk.

Orthostatic hypotension (OH)

→ A ↓ in SBP ≥ 20 mmHg or DBP ≥ 10 mmHg within 3 minutes after standing from supine state

→ If the reduction in BP occurs after 3 minutes of standing: vasovagal syncope, and sympathetic dysfunction.

→ Causes includes:

- Cardiac: MI, aortic valve stenosis, dehydration, vasodilatation due to fever, etc.
- Neurogenic: Neuropathy, parkinsonism, etc.
- Drugs: Diuretics, alfa blockers, calcium channel blockers, Insulin, tricyclic antidepressants, levodopa.

→ Prevalence is more in the elderly population

→ Diabetes and hypertension are associated with higher deaths in OH.

→ Diastolic OH indicates higher risk of vascular deaths.

White coat hypertension

→ Office BP ≥ 140/90 mmHg and a 24 hour ABPM (home) reading < 130/80 mmHg.

→ Occurs in 15-30% patients.

→ More common in females, elderly, nonsmokers, and recently diagnosed hypertensives.

→ ABPM is indicated to diagnose White coat hypertension when: the clinic (office) BP ≥ 140/90 mmHg on ≥ 3 different visits, ≥ 2 home BP readings are < 140/90 mmHg, no target organ damage due to hypertension.

→ Once confirmed of White coat hypertension, the patients should be rechecked in a 3-6 months period and then annually by ABPM to discover true sustained hypertension.

Resistant hypertension

→ Uncontrolled hypertension in a patient taking at least 3 classes of antihypertensive medications, out of which one is a diuretic.

Hypertension in pregnancy

→ MC disorder complicating pregnancies.

→ Affects 5-10% of all pregnancies.

→ Ideally diagnosed by ABPM, but most commonly detected by standard clinic BP determinations.

→ Can be mild (SBP- 140-159 mmHg and/or DBP- 90-109 mmHg), and severe (BP ≥ 160/110 mmHg).

→ Pre-existing hypertension: hypertension present before the pregnancy or before 20 weeks of gestation or is present even after 6 weeks postpartum.

→ Gestational hypertension: develops after 20 weeks of gestation and improves within 6 weeks postpartum. It is a type of secondary hypertension only.

→ Pre-eclampsia: Gestational hypertension + proteinuria > 0.3 g/day.

→ Eclampsia: pre-eclampsia + GTC seizures.

→ Complications: Maternal mortality (9%), premature delivery, HELLP syndrome (haemolysis, elevated liver enzymes, low platelets).

Classification of hypertension (2017 ACC/AHA guidelines)

Normal	⇨	SBP < 120 mmHg **and** DBP < 80 mmHg
Elevated	⇨	SBP 120-129 mmHg **and** DBP < 80 mmHG
Stage I hypertension	⇨	SBP 130-139 mmHg **or** DBP 80-89 mmHG
Stage II hypertension	⇨	SBP ≥ 140 mmHG **or** DBP ≥ 90 mmHg.

References

- Jean-Pierre Barral D.O. (UK), MRO (F), Alain Croibier D.O., MRO (F), in Visceral Vascular Manipulations, 2011;ScienceDirect:Circulatory physiology.
- Cardiol Clin. 2010 November; 28 (4): 571-586. doi:10.1016/j.ccl.2010.07.006 Principles and techniques of blood pressure measurement.

- Hypertension. 2019;73:e35–e66.Measurement of Blood Pressure in Humans;A Scientific Statement From the American Heart Association.
- The Art and Science of Cardiac Physical Examination by Narasimhan Ranganathan.
- MJAFI 2003; 59: 51·52 Technique of Blood Pressure Measurement.
- Clinical methods in cardiology by B Soma Raju.
- Clinical examination in cardiology by B N Vijay Raghav Rao 2nd edition.
- (Journal of the American Association for Laboratory Animal Science Vol 57, No 1 January 2018 Pages 64–69 Comparison of Direct and Indirect Methods of Measuring Arterial Blood Pressure in Healthy Male Rhesus Macaques (Macaca mulatta).
- Nursing2004, Volume 34, Number 11 Taking blood pressure accurately.
- Z Kardiol. 1996;85 Suppl 3:92-8.Automated blood pressure measurement in special situations: patients with chronic atrial fibrillation or chronic aortic regurgitation.
- Nursing and Midwifery Research Journal, Vol-4, No. 4, October 2008 A study to evaluate the clinical value of Hill's sign in the assessment of aortic regurgitation.
- Calif Med. 1957 Sep; 87 (3): 166–167 DETERMINING BLOOD PRESSURE IN INFANTS—Use of the Flush Technique.
- European society of cardiology Vol. 17, N° 22 - 18 Sep 2019 Hypertension in pregnancy.
- Cleve Clin J Med. 2010 May; 77 (5): 298–306. doi:10.3949/ccjm.77a.09118. Preventing and treating orthostatic hypotension: As easy as A, B, C.
- Hypertension. 2013;62:982–987 White-Coat Hypertension; New Insights From Recent Studies.

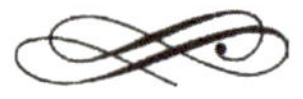

CHAPTER

4 Jugular Venous Pulse

Jugular venous pulse (and pressure) (JVP) is a very important part of the cardiovascular system examination but unfortunately it is neglected by us most of the time.

It gives information about the cardiac filling pressure.

A careful examination of the JVP can give ideas about the hemodynamic information of the right side of the heart.

Central venous pressure (CVP) = Mean right atrial pressure = Right end diastolic pressure in the absence of TR.

CVP is determined by an invasive method with a manometer. The bedside clinical examination for JVP can give ideas about the CVP.

The CVP and JVP are expressed in cmH_2O (1 mmHg = 1.36 cmH_2O).

The external reference point

Before measuring the JVP, we should have a reference point with respect to which we judge the JVP.

Reference point means a point in the CVS at which the CVP is strictly regulated.

This point is the centre of the right atrium or the phlebostatic axis. But we cannot go to the right atrium to measure this pressure clinically. Hence, the corresponding external reference point is the sternal angle which lies approximately 5 cm above the centre of the right atrium. The starting and the endpoint of the JVP are the phlebostatic axis and the topmost venous column in the neck, respectively.

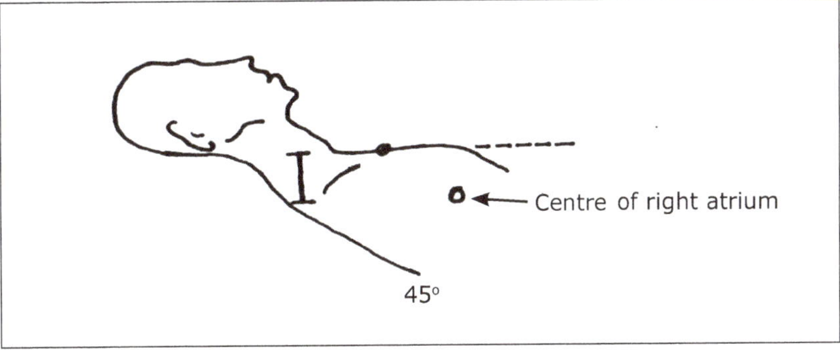

Fig. 4.1: External reference point.

Site of JVP

The right internal jugular vein (RIJV) is preferred for JVP because it has no valves and is connected in a straight line to the SVC. Hence, it gives an accurate estimate of the right atrial pressure(RAP).

The left internal jugular vein drains into the left innominate vein but not in a straight line.

The external jugular veins (EJV) are not chosen because: (1) they join the SVC at right angles, (2) they pass through several fascial planes and can be easily compressed by external pressure, (3) they go into vasoconstriction with sympathetic stimulation.

Sometimes however, there may be difficulty in differentiating the JVP from the carotid artery pulsations.

Table 4.1: The differentiating points between the two pulsations

CAROTID ARTERY PULSE	JUGULAR VENOUS PULSE
Pulse seen internal to Sternocleidomastoid (SM) muscle	Seen inside a triangle formed by the 2 heads of the SM muscle and the clavicle
Strikes the palpating finger	It is better visible
Seen as a thrusting outward pulsation	Inward movement
Exhibits a single upstroke	Has 2 peaks and 2 troughs per cardiac cycle
Does not change with posture or respiration	Decreases with upright posture and inspiration
Compression does not obliterate the pulse	Compression at the root of the neck abolishes the pulse

Technique to measure JVP

The patient's thorax and neck is exposed and he/she is directed to rest the head on a pillow (if required) without acute angulation of the head with respect to the neck.

The JVP can also be seen by throwing a tangential light over the neck.

For most of the cardiac disorders, the patient is asked to lie in a 45^0 inclined supine position. If the expected JVP appears to be very high, a more inclined position of 60^0 or even 90^0 may be needed to make the IJV pulsations visible. Contrary to this, if the JVP is less, we may need to give a 30^0 inclined posture to the patient.

If required, one may lift the patient's legs to make the pulsations more prominent by increasing the venous return.

Coordinating the venous pulsations with the cardiac cycle can be done by simultaneous palpation of the left carotid pulse.

Now after all this is done, we see the venous column and try to locate the uppermost level of it.

Two horizontal lines are made (in relation to the floor) with the help of wooden or plastic scales. One from the upper level of the venous column and the other from the sternal angle. The distance between these two lines plus 5 cm (sternal angle to centre of right atrium distance) gives us the Jugular venous pressure in cmH_2O. The normal jugular venous pressure should not exceed 9 cmH_2O (7 mmHg).

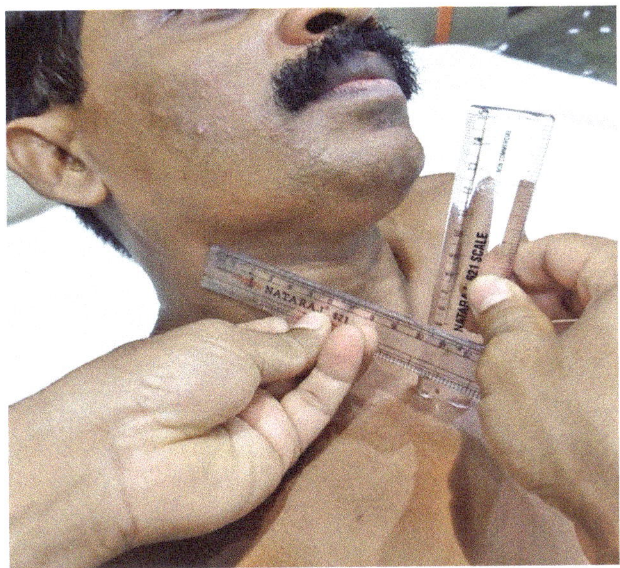

Fig. 4.2: Technique to measure JVP.

One alternative method to roughly estimate the venous pressure is to examine the veins of the dorsum of the hand. With the patient sitting or at 30^0 inclined position, the arm is slowly raised from the dependent position.

If the venous pressure is within normal limits, the veins collapse as the hand reaches the level of the sternal angle. This method is useful for cases where the CVP is exceptionally high and the venous column is above the angle of the mandible even in sitting posture.

Causes of raised JVP:

→ Non pulsatile: SVC obstruction (bilaterally raised JVP), Innominate vein thrombosis (unilaterally raised JVP)

→ Pulsatile: CCF, constrictive pericarditis, cardiac tamponade, TR, TS, cor pulmonale, fluid overload, etc.

Causes of decreased JVP:

→ Hypovolemic shock, Addison's disease.

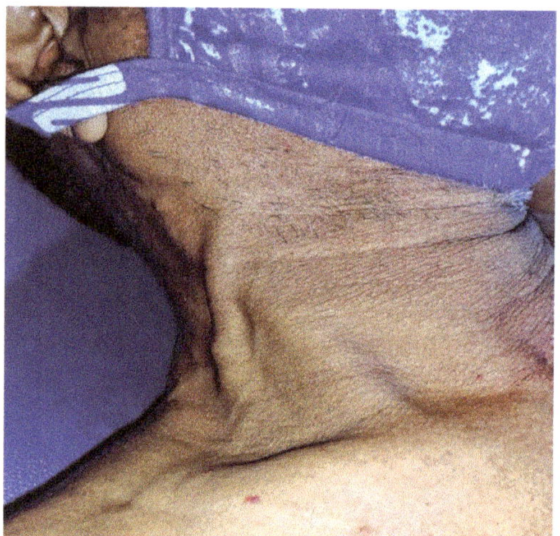

Fig. 4.3: A case of raised JVP.

> **NOTE**
>
> The JVP is useful to differentiate the etiology of edema with breathlessness. For instance, edema caused by ↓ oncotic pressure states like liver disease, nephrotic syndrome or GIT causes has ↓ intravascular volume, and hence a flat JVP, i.e; low venous pressure.
>
> In edema due to CVS disorders, the JVP is raised due to ↑ RAP s/o ↑ pulmonary artery wedge pressure.

Normal JVP waves

The normal JVP has 2 positive waves - a and v, and 2 negative waves - x and y.

Sometimes additional waves can be obtained namely the positive waves c and h.

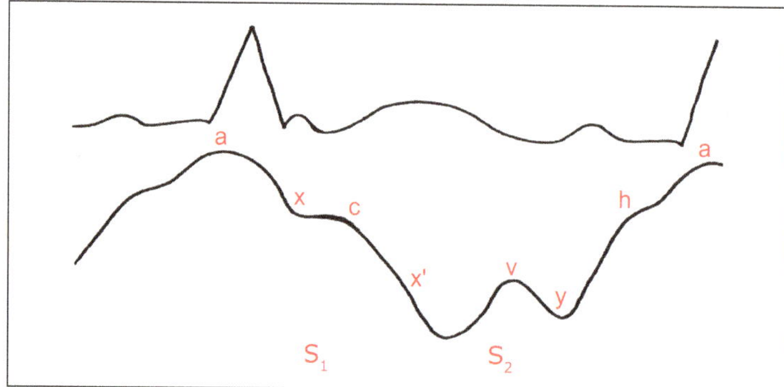

Fig. 4.4: Normal Jugular venous wave pattern.

a wave

→ 1st positive wave

→ Occurs due to atrial contraction and just before the carotid pulse and S1

→ Coincides with S4

→ Larger than v wave

x descent

→ It occurs due to the pressure fall while right atrium starts relaxing (which means that ventricular systole has begun) (please keep in mind about the cardiac events that takes place in cycle while reading JVP)

→ Starts at early systole

→ Finishes before S2

→ Usually larger than the y descent

c wave

→ As the ventricular systole begins, the ventricular pressure starts increasing above the atrial pressure leading to closure of the tricuspid valve

→ During isovolumetric contraction, the closed tricuspid valves start bulging upwards that creates a positive wave called the c wave.

→ c wave indicates the T1 component of the S1

x' descent

→ During the early phase of ventricular systole, we get the x descent as explained above. But as the atrial relaxation continues, the atrial pressure falls further leading to a downward pull on the tricuspid valve which produces this x' descent.

→ Hence, it is noteworthy that the x descent is interrupted by a positive c wave followed by the x' descent in sequence.

→ x' occurs along with the radial pulse

v wave

→ As the ventricular systole advances with a closed tricuspid valve, the right atrium continues to receive blood from the larger veins leading to a rise in the right atrial pressure which forms the v wave.

→ The v wave terminates the x descent

→ It is the 2nd positive wave in the JVP waveforms.

→ It starts in late systole and terminates in early phases of diastole, coinciding with carotid upstroke.

→ The v wave peaks after S2

y descent

→ It occurs during early ventricular diastole when the tricuspid valve opens with flow of blood from the atrium to the ventricle with a fall in right atrial pressure

→ The early phase of the y descent is due to the rapid filling of the RV

→ It terminates after the S2

h wave

→ First coined by Arthur D Hirschfelder (hence h wave).

→ It occurs during the passive RV filling phase in diastole just before the next a wave, especially if the heart rate is slow.

NOTE

Prominent x and y descent → during inspiration.

Prominent v wave and diminished a wave → during expiration.

We use the x and y descent to time the venous pulse as the x descent coincides with the carotid and radial pulse.

ABNORMALITIES OF THE JVP WAVES

Abnormalities of a wave

(1) Prominent a waves

→ Increased resistance to ventricular filling: Tricuspid stenosis, tricuspid atresia, right atrial myxoma.

→ Decreased RV compliance: RV hypertrophy, ischemia, acute pulmonary embolism, RV infiltration, RV fibrosis.

→ Bernheim's effect: Aortic stenosis, severe left ventricular hypertrophy.

(Bernheim's effect: decreased RV filling due to shift of septum to the right due to a left heart pathology leading to RV failure)

(2) Cannon a waves

→ Atria and ventricles contract without any co-ordination

→ Hence atria may contract when the tricuspid valve is closed leading to a cannon(giant) a wave

→ Regular cannon a waves: Junctional rhythm, isorhythmic AV dissociation

→ Irregular cannon a waves: Complete AV block, ventricular pacemaker, ventricular tachycardia

(3) Absent a waves

→ Ineffective and disorganised atrial contraction and relaxation: Atrial fibrillation

→ Fusion of the a and v waves: Sinus tachycardia

Abnormalities of x descent

(1) Absent x descent

→ Tricuspid regurgitation: Leads to an early rise of the RA pressure resulting in loss of x descent. The x descent loss may also be because of the development of early systolic v waves(or cv waves) followed by the y descent.

→ Atrial fibrillation: No Starling effect (RV dysfunction).

→ Bernheim effect: MR

→ ↓RV contractility: RV infarct, RVF in pulmonary hypertension.

(2) Prominent x descent

→ Cardiac tamponade and constrictive pericarditis: Vigorous RV contraction

→ Atrial septal defect: Overload of the RV.

Abnormalities of the v wave

(1) Prominent v wave

→ Tricuspid regurgitation: There is filling of the RA from the great veins during ventricular systole as well as retrograde filling due to TV leak. The x descent is obliterated by the tall v waves or cv waves (as described above), also termed as Lancisi sign.

→ Large ASD, Gerbode defect (LV to RA type VSD): Vena caval venous return plus the L→R shunting of blood increasing the RA pressure.

→ AV fistula (hemodialysis patients): Due to shunting of blood to the venous system.

(2) Decreased v wave

→ Hypovolemic state

→ Use of nitrates (venodilators).

Abnormalities of the y descent

(1) Slow y descent

→ Impedance to RA outflow: Tricuspid stenosis

→ Resistance to RV filling: Severe RV hypertrophy

→ Shortened diastole: Tachycardia

→ Compromised RV filling due to raised intrapericardial pressure: Cardiac tamponade (y descent may even be absent).

(2) Rapid y descent

→ ↑RAP and rapid emptying: Tricuspid regurgitation, constrictive pericarditis (Friedreich sign), restrictive cardiomyopathy.

Kussmaul sign

→ Normally, with inspiration the RAP and JV pressure falls due to negative intrapleural pressure that causes more flow of blood from the right heart to the lungs.

→ The absence of this decrease in JV pressure or a paradoxical increase is known as Kussmaul sign.

→ One hypothesis about the mechanism causing Kussmaul sign is a non-compliant pericardium which fails to redistribute the increased venous return during inspiration. This causes a rise in the RAP more than the fall in the pleural pressure causing a rise in the JV pressure with inspiration.

→ Causes of Kussmaul sign: Severe right heart failure (MC), constrictive pericarditis, right ventricular MI, severe TR, restrictive cardiomyopathy.

Hepatojugular reflux (HJR)

→ It is one more method of detecting the venous pressure.

→ This method is useful in patients with right heart failure who have either normal or borderline raised JV pressure.

→ The test is done by applying a firm and sustained pressure over the right upper part of the abdomen for about 10-15 seconds with the patient breathing normally.

→ This increases the venous return from the abdomen towards the heart.

→ A failing heart cannot handle this increased venous return and the JVP rises throughout the sustained abdominal pressure.

→ Do not ask the patient to perform Valsalva as this would nullify the venous return by increasing the intrathoracic pressure.

→ In the normal state, the JVP rises only transiently and not > 1 cmH_2O and returns back to the normal.

→ However, with right heart failure, the JVP rises by > 3 cmH_2O and remains elevated throughout the period of abdominal compression.

→ A positive test also indicates a PCWP of 15 mmHg or more (equivalent to left atrial pressure), if there is no right heart infarction.

→ Other conditions with positive HJR are: constrictive pericarditis, restrictive cardiomyopathy, and TR.

JVP in some particular diseases

(1) JVP in pulmonary hypertension

→ Prominent v wave: due to ↑ RVEDP

→ Decreased x' descent: only if there is an associated ↓ in RV systolic function.

(2) JVP in post cardiac surgery patients

→ In post cardiopulmonary bypass surgery patients, the RA loses its function as a capacitance chamber and behaves like a conduit only because of edema and scarring.

→ Steep y descent: due to transmission of the diastolic flow velocity at tricuspid level to the SVC

(3) JVP in SVC obstruction

→ With total obstruction, the venous pressure is markedly elevated with distension of the arm veins.

→ No pulsations in the JVP are visible.

(4) JVP in tricuspid stenosis (TS)

→ May be elevated or sometimes normal in very mild TS or when the patient is on therapy with diuretics.

→ Prominent a wave: due to ↑ resistance to ventricular filling, which transmits most of the atrial contraction pressure to the neck veins.

→ Larger than normal v waves: but smaller than the a waves (except in AFib where v waves becomes the only positive wave).

→ Slow y descent: due to impedance to RA outflow.

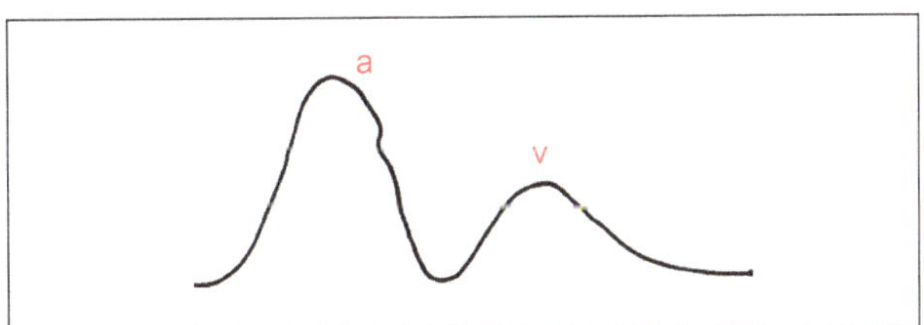

Fig. 4.5: Prominent 'a' wave in tricuspid stenosis.

(5) JVP in tricuspid regurgitation(TR)

→ Prominent a wave: only if there is associated PAH or the TR is acute in onset.

→ Absent x descent: due to early rise of the RA pressure.

→ Very prominent v wave: due to filling of the RA from the vena cavae and the TV leak (retrograde filling).

→ Steep y descent: due to ↑ RAP and rapid emptying.

→ Prominent h wave

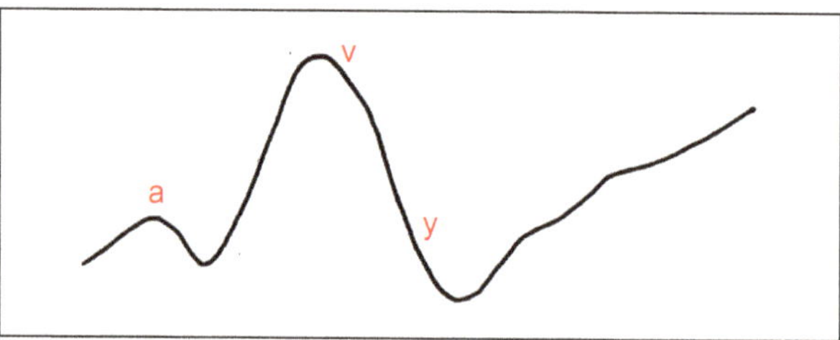

Fig. 4.6: Absent 'x' descent with rapid 'y' descent with prominent 'v' waves in Tricuspid regurgitation.

(6) JVP in pulmonary stenosis (PS)

→ PS in the long run can lead to RV failure and development of TR. Hence, the JVP findings may be normal or similar to those found in TR (described above).

→ However, most of the times PS may be clinically confused with a small VSD or TOF. The presence of a prominent a wave indicates an intact interventricular septum and rules out VSD of TOF clinically.

(7) JVP in mitral stenosis (MS)

→ The JVP in MS is a bit tricky because many times MS may occur in association with TS or an ASD (Lutembacher syndrome) or may lead to the development of PAH.

→ Prominent a wave: if there is associated PAH or TS, else normal.

→ Absent x descent: if MS patient develops AFib, else normal.

→ Prominent v wave: if TR or PAH develops, else normal.

→ Steep y descent: if associated TR develops due to PAH, else normal.

→ Slow y descent: if associated TS present, else normal.

(8) JVP in mitral regurgitation (MR)

→ JVP in MR is more or less normal until the development of complications like PAH, TR or associated conditions like HCM or CAD.

→ Prominent a wave: if there is PAH or associated HCM.

→ Prominent v waves: if PAH or TR present

→ Steep y descent: if TR.

(9) JVP in aortic stenosis (AS)

→ Prominent a waves: due to Bernheim's effect.

(10) JVP in aortic regurgitation (AR)

→ Prominent a waves: due to Bernheim's effect sometimes.

→ Rest of the JVP findings depend on the presence or absence of associated lesions like PAH, dissection, RV failure etc.

(11) JVP in Ebstein's anomaly

→ In Ebstein's anomaly, there is abnormal downward displacement of the tricuspid valve leading to atrialization of the basal RV and varying degrees of TR.

→ The RA increases in size with increased capacitance.

→ Hence, the JVP shows all the features of TR but may not be reflected properly due to the increased RA capacitance.

(12) JVP in atrial septal defect (ASD)

→ Prominent x descent: due to a strong Starling effect as a result of an increased RV volume.

→ Sometimes x'=y descent in very large sized ASD due to equalization of pressures in both the atria.

→ Prominent v wave: due to overloaded RA.

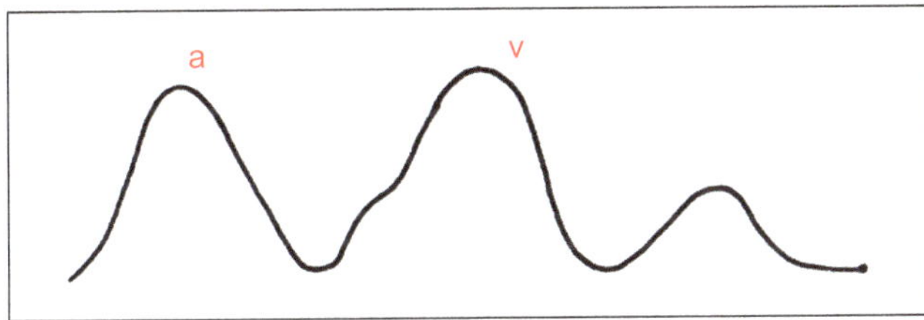

Fig. 4.7: Prominent 'a' and 'v' waves in ASD.

(13) JVP in ventricular septal defect (VSD)

→ Normal a wave

→ Prominent v wave: especially in Gerbode defect (LV to RA defect) due to raised RA pressure.

(14) JVP in cardiomyopathies

→ Hypertrophic cardiomyopathy: Prominent a wave

→ Endomyocardial fibrosis: Prominent a wave, Prominent v wave, and steep y descent.

(15) JVP in Cardiac tamponade

→ It is a state of total diastolic restriction

- → It is a condition where the heart is under tremendous intrapericardial pressure from all sides as if encased in a hard and tight box.
- → During diastole, no blood can enter the heart due to the surrounding pressure.
- → The only period when blood can enter the heart is the systole when the ventricles have the smallest size.
- → x' descent is the only recordable wave during inspiration.
- → Absent y descent: due to compromised RV filling due to raised intrapericardial pressure.
- → However, there are few conditions where the patient can present to you with a normal JVP despite having cardiac tamponade like post- or perioperative tamponade, Intradialysis state, tamponade due to multiple trauma, LV tamponade after heart surgery, diuretic therapy, etc. The basic underlying pathology common to all these mentioned causes of low pressure tamponade is hypovolemia/blood loss.

(16) JVP in constrictive pericarditis

- → Rapid y descent: due to ↑ RAP and rapid emptying.
- → In some atypical cases there may be a dominant x' descent when the RV early diastolic pressure is high with little difference between the RA and RV pressures leading to a poor y descent.

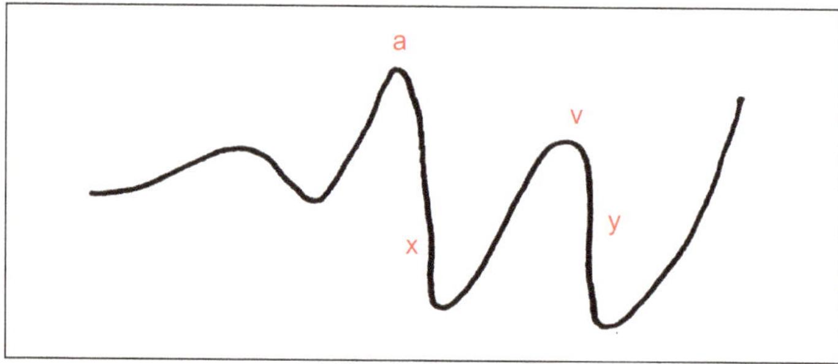

Fig. 4.8: Prominent 'x', 'y' descent with prominent 'a' and 'v' waves in Constrictive pericarditis.

(17) JVP in cardiac arrhythmias

- → Sinus rhythm: a wave followed by v wave normally.

  a wave along with S1 indicates a normal PR interval. a wave coincides with P wave and v wave coincides with the QRS complex of the Electrocardiogram. The number of a and v waves should be equal normally.
- → 1^0 AV block: a wave followed by v wave, but a wave coming well before S1.
- → Mobitz type I AV block (Wenckebach phenomenon):

  Gradual prolonging of the a-v interval followed by a sudden absence of v wave or S1.

→ Mobitz type II AV block: Preserved a-v interval with sudden loss of v wave.

→ 2^0 AV block: 2 a waves: 1 v wave or S1

→ 3^0 AV block: Irregular cannon a waves with the number of a waves > v waves or S1, without coordination.

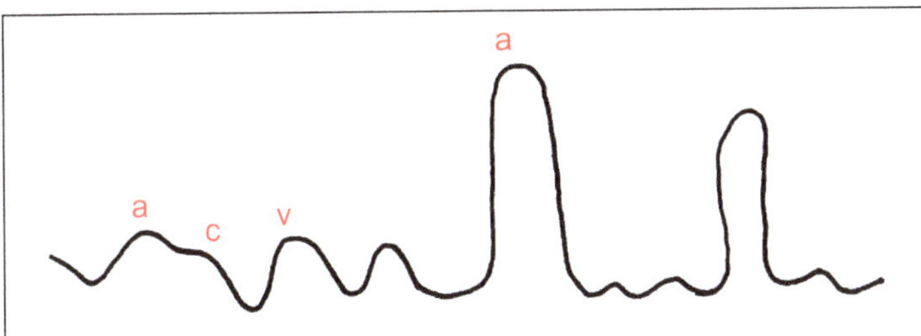

Fig. 4.9: Irregular cannon 'a' waves in complete AV block.

→ Junctional rhythm: Regular cannon a waves

→ Ventricular tachycardia: Irregular cannon a waves

→ Atrial tachycardia: Normal a and v waves.

References

- Journal, Indian Academy of Clinical Medicine Vol. 1, No. 3 October-December 2000 Jugular Venous Pulse : An Appraisal.
- APIINDIA chapter 195 Back to Bedside Basics - Pulse, Blood Pressure and Jugular Venous Pulse.
- The art and science of cardiac physical examination by Ranganathan.
- Postgrad Med J: first published as 10.1136/pgmj.33.382.389 on 1 August 1957 THE JUGULAR VENOUS PULSE.
- Clinical methods: The history, physical, and laboratory examinations.3rd edition Chapter 19 The Jugular Venous Pressure and Pulse Contour.
- Clinical examination in cardiology 2nd edition by B N Vijaya Raghawa Rao.
- JAMA. 1953;152(6):551. doi:10.1001/jama.1953.03690060067028AORTIC STENOSIS AND BERNHEIM'S SYNDROME.
- Southern Medical Journal • Volume 100, Number 10, October 2007 Jugular Venous Pulse: Window into the Right Heart.
- Singh N, Chadha DS, Bharadwaj P, Agarwal N. Adolf Kussmaul and Kussmaul's sign. J Pract Cardiovasc Sci 2015;1:128-9.
- Houston and Stevens. Hypertrophic Cardiomyopathy: A Review. Clinical Medicine Insights: Cardiology 2014:8(S1) 53–65 doi: 10.4137/CMC.S15717.

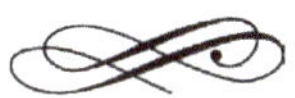

CHAPTER

5 Inspection of the Anterior Chest and Precordium (CVS)

Just like the other components of cardiovascular system examination, inspection of the precordium is as useful. A proper inspection of the precordium can give as valuable information as can be obtained from some noninvasive studies.

The components of inspection must include

(1) Looking for the shape of the chest, skin lesions, abnormalities of the breast, and abnormal veins over the chest.

(2) Any precordial bulging

(3) CVS pulsations like apical impulse, pulsations in pulmonary and aortic areas, epigastric pulsations etc.

SHAPE OF THE CHEST

To examine the shape of the chest, the patient should lie in a supine position on the bed, sometimes inclined slightly (not > 30^0 elevated).

The chest is visualized in a tangential manner, first from the foot end and then from the right side.

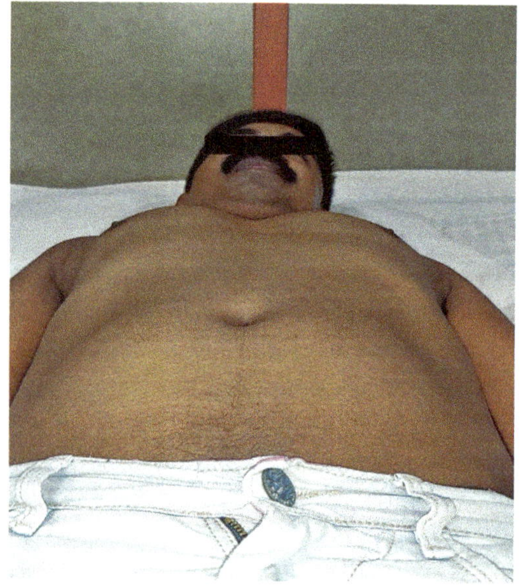

Fig. 5.1: Tangential examination of the chest from the foot end.

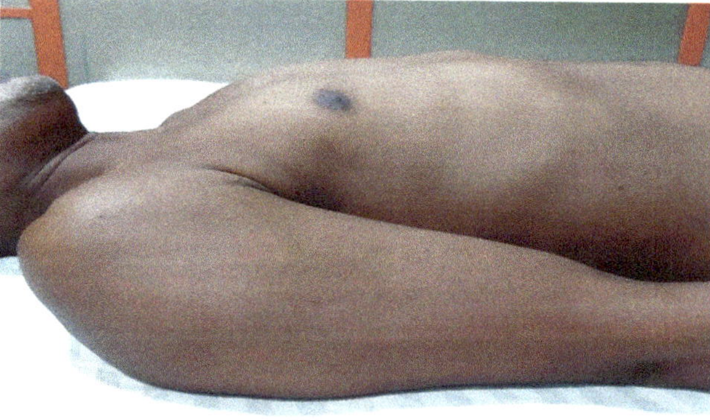

Fig. 5.2: Tangential examination of the chest from the patient's right side.

One can also use a torch light beam across the precordium for better visibility.

A normal chest is symmetrical with a transverse diameter/anteroposterior diameter ratio of approximately 7:5.

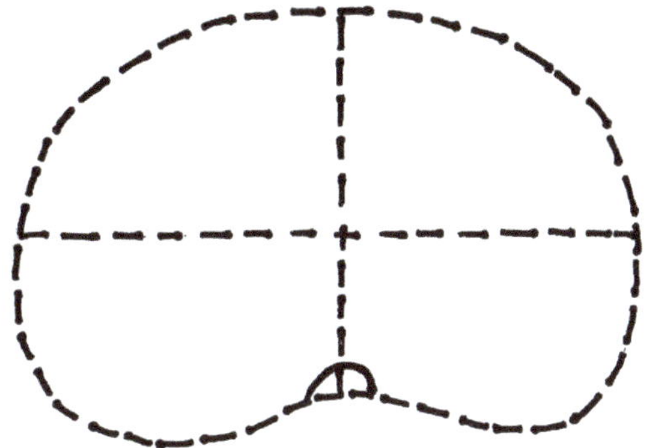

Fig. 5.3: Normal adult chest cross-sectional diagram.

Pectus excavatum

→ Also called funnel chest or sunken chest

→ Constitutes > 87% of all chest deformities

→ There is posteriorly displaced sternum

→ M:F = 3:1

→ Associated scoliosis may be found in upto 29%

→ Common cardiac diseases found in association with pectus excavatum are ↓ stroke volume and cardiac output, MVP (15%), arrhythmias (1^0 heart block, bundle branch block, WPW syndrome).

→ Common in Marfan's syndrome, Ehlers-danlos syndrome, Straight back syndrome.

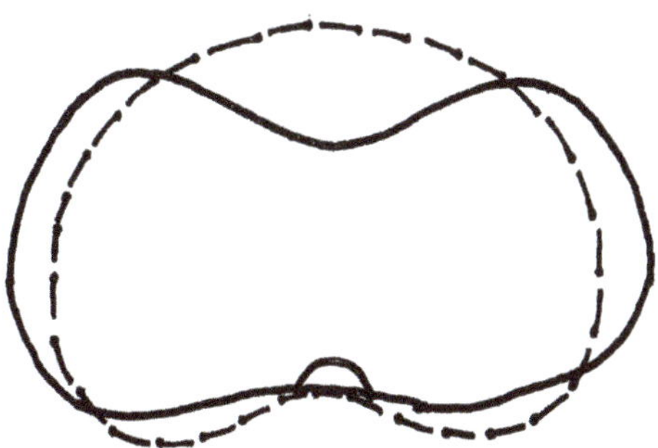

Fig. 5.4: Pectus excavatum.

Pectus carinatum

→ Also called pigeon breast

→ Abnormal protrusion of the sternum and costal cartilages

→ M:F = 2:1

→ Associated with Marfan's syndrome, Noonan syndrome, Rickets.

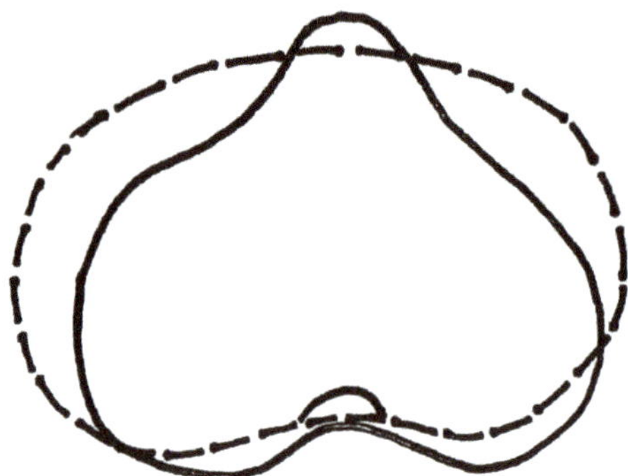

Fig. 5.5: Pectus carinatum.

Barrel shaped chest

→ The anteroposterior diameter of the chest is increased, ribs are more horizontal, angle of Louis is prominent, and the chest is inflated.

→ Commonly seen in COPD

→ It interferes with the cardiac examinations and heart sounds.

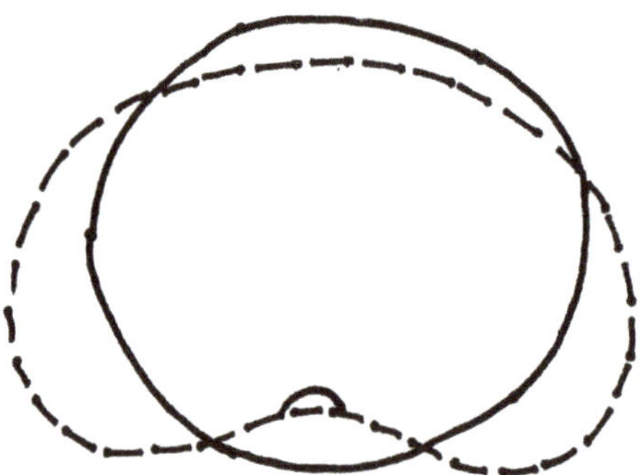

Fig. 5.6: Barrel shaped chest.

Shield chest

→ Broad chest with widely spaced nipples

→ Seen in Turner's syndrome and Noonan syndrome.

Straight back syndrome

→ Loss of thoracic kyphosis → reduced AP diameter of the chest → compression or "pancaking" of the heart and great vessels so as to appear enlarged (described earlier in general examination).

SKIN OVER THE CHEST

Erythema marginatum

→ Nonpruritic macular rash with erythematous and serpiginous border, about 0.5 cm in diameter, and usually located over the trunk and inner aspect of the proximal parts of the limbs.

→ Characteristic of Rheumatic fever.

Café au lait spots (macules)

→ Neurofibromatosis

Flushing

→ Carcinoid syndrome

BREAST ABNORMALITIES

Gynecomastia

→ Development of female-like breasts in males can be seen in conditions like Klinefelter syndrome, and as adverse effects of drugs like digitalis and spironolactone.

Hypomastia in females

→ Seen in MVP

Widely spaced nipples

→ Turner's syndrome, Noonan syndrome.

Abnormal vessels over the chest

→ Dilated veins over the chest may indicate SVC obstruction

→ Suzman sign: dilated collateral arteries seen near the scapulae in coarctation of aorta, especially on bending forward with the arms hanging.

BULGING OF THE PRECORDIUM

Cardiac causes

→ Pericardial effusion: bulging of only intercostal spaces (ICS) (no rib involvement).

→ Ventricular enlargement (usually RV): bulging of ICS and the ribs.

→ Ventricular aneurysm (long standing): localized bulging (rarely).

→ Large ASD with PAH: left precordial bulge.

Respiratory causes

→ Pleural effusion

→ Bronchogenic carcinoma

→ Mediastinal growth

Skeletal causes

→ Kyphoscoliosis

→ Rickets

APICAL IMPULSE

Defined as the lateral most and lowest point of systolic outward motion seen on the chest wall in early systole followed by a very mild medial retraction in later part of the systole.

During the isovolumetric contraction phase, the LV moves anteriorly slightly and also rotates in counterclockwise direction along its long axis which causes the apex to make contact with the left chest wall causing the early systolic thrust.

The recoil of the LV after completing the ejection process in late systole causes the medial retraction.

The medial retraction reflects that the apical impulse is formed by the LV. It is better seen than felt. Usually checked in lateral decubitus position after palpating the apical impulse and keeping the finger in place we try to see the medial (and also lateral) retraction.

If this inward retraction occurs lateral to the apical impulse, it is called a lateral retraction.

Lateral retraction is an abnormal finding and indicates that the apical impulse is formed by an enlarged RV.

Location

→ 5th intercostal space in midclavicular line or within 10 cm to the left of midsternal line.

→ It is usually checked in sitting posture.

Area

→ Not > 2.5-3.0 cm in diameter.

→ Usually measures two fingers in breadth horizontally and occupies 1 intercostal space in vertical dimension.

→ Area > 3.0 cm in diameter is called a wide area apex.

Hyperdynamic apex impulse

→ When the amplitude of the impulse is increased.

→ Indicates a diastolic volume overload state like beri beri, AV fistula, thyrotoxicosis, Paget's disease, pregnancy, anemia etc.

→ Cardiac causes include MR, AR, VSD, PDA etc.

→ The large volume is ejected with great force and velocity as per Starling's law leading to increased amplitude of the impulse.

→ One can put the head of the stethoscope over the apical impulse and then see its rigorous movements due to the hyperdynamic impulse.

Sustained (heaving) apical impulse

→ Amplitude + duration of the impulse is increased.

→ To detect the duration of the impulse, we palpate the impulse in sitting or left lateral position and simultaneously auscultate the cardiac sounds (S1 and S2) in the left 3rd or 4th intercostal space.

→ The normal impulse rises and falls quickly along with the S1.

→ If the apical impulse is felt to recede by the palpating hand simultaneously with the S2, we say that the apical impulse is sustained (> 50% of the systole).

→ It indicates an ↑ in the LV mass and volume and is usually also seen with LV dysfunction.

→ However, the sustained impulse signifies a sustained ↑ in the LV wall tension due to volume or pressure overload that causes the LV mass to rise.

→ Can be seen in conditions like AS, severe hypertension, LV dysfunction, etc.

ABNORMALITIES OF THE APICAL IMPULSE

Invisible apical impulse

→ DCM, pericardial effusion, poor cardiac contractions due to MI, heart behind a rib, etc.

→ Large breasts, emphysema, thick chest, etc.

Double apical impulse

→ HOCM (characteristic). Consists of an atrial beat due to ↑ atrial contraction filling the LV and the second beat due to sudden obstruction at the LVOT level due to SAM (systolic anterior motion of the mitral valve) (can sometimes be associated with triple apical beat also when there is an associated palpable S4).

→ MVP

→ Post MI LV dyskinesia

Downward displacement of the apical impulse

→ Aortic aneurysm

→ Mediastinal growth

Upward displacement of the apical impulse

→ Ascites

→ Tumor of the abdomen

→ Pregnancy

Right sided apical impulse

→ Dextrocardia

Apical impulse shifted down and out

→ LV enlargement, e.g; AR

Apical impulse shifted out (laterally)

→ RV enlargement

Apical impulse diffuse

→ Thin subject

→ Hyperdynamic states

→ Regurgitant valve lesions

→ L→R shunts

→ Complete heart block

→ HOCM

Lateral retraction of apical impulse

→ RVH

→ Skoda's sign: systolic retraction and diastolic elevation seen in adhesive pericarditis

→ Broadbent's sign: Indrawing of 11th and 12th ribs with intercostal space narrowing posteriorly seen in adhesive pericarditis.

Pulsations in the right 2nd intercostal space (aortic area)

→ This area corresponds to the ascending aorta

→ Pulsations in this area are seen in ascending aortic aneurysm, aortic dilatation, severe AR.

Pulsations in the left 2nd or 3rd intercostal space (pulmonary area and Erb's area)

→ Pulmonary trunk at pulmonary area

→ Infundibulum or RVOT at Erb's area

→ Pulsations in these areas are seen in pulmonary artery dilatation in PDA or ASD, PAH in MS, descending thoracic aneurysm, etc.

→ Left 4th or 5th intercostal spaces correspond to the RV inflow portion.

Pulsations in sternoclavicular (SC) joints

→ Right aortic arch (Right SC joint)

→ Dissection of aorta, aneurysm of aorta

Suprasternal pulsations

→ Hyperdynamic circulation

→ Atherosclerotic dilatation of the aorta

→ Syphilitic aortitis

→ Innominate artery flexion

→ Anomalous right subclavian artery

Pulsations at the left parasternal area (LPA)

→ Pulsations at the left side of the sternum mainly between the 3rd and 6th ribs are related to RV pathology.

→ Causes could be:

- RV pressure overload (PAH) or RV volume overload (ASD)
- Anterior displacement of the RV due to pressure from behind (Enlarged LA due to severe MS)

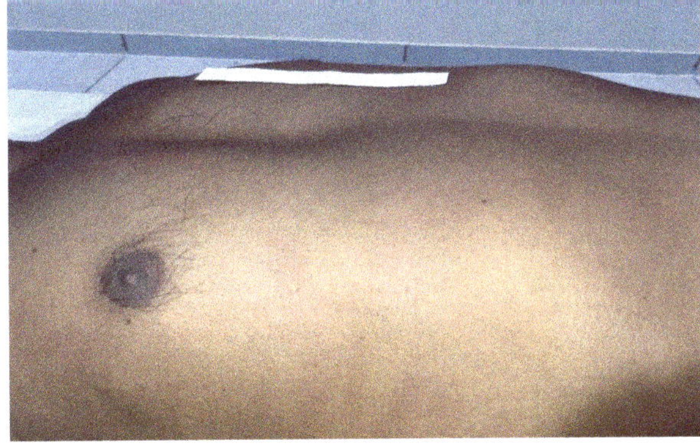

Fig. 5.7: LPA pulsations visualised by putting a piece of paper over the chest.

- Severe MR causing enlarged LA during systole that pushes the RV forward
- Aneurysm of the LV that causes abnormal anterior movement during contraction.

→ LPA pulsations can be better detected visually by putting a light object like a rectangular piece of paper or a pen over the chest and looking for their spontaneous pulsatile movements.

Epigastric pulsations

→ Aortic pulsations

→ Liver pulsations (TS or TR)

→ RVH in MS

Subxiphoid pulsations

→ Very specific for RV impulse.

→ Palpated with the hand over the epigastrium and the fingers facing the head of the patient

→ If the pulsations hit the fingertips then they are RV impulses. If the pulsations hit the palm then they are abdominal aortic pulsations.

Pulsations in the right lower chest (4th intercostal space)

→ RA impulses in severe TR

References

- Chest wall anomalies: pectus excavatum and pectus carinatum.Michael J. Goretsky, Robert E. Kelly, Daniel Croitoru, Donald Nuss. Adolesc Med 15 (2004) 455-471.
- Pectus excavatum, pectus carinatum and other forms of thoracic deformities. J Indian Assoc Pediatr Surg/Jul-Sept 2005/Vol 10/ Issue 3. A K Saxena.
- N Engl J Med 1983; 309:1230-1232 DOI: 10.1056/NEJM198311173092007 Hypomastia and Mitral-Valve Prolapse — Evidence of a Linked Embryologic and Mesenchymal Dysplasia.
- Br Heart J. 1947 Jul; 9(3): 185-212. COARCTATION OF THE AORTA Maurice Campbell and S. Suzman.
- A textbook of symptoms and physical signs by Rustom Jal Vakil and Aspi F Golwalla.
- Erciyes Med J 2019; 41(2): 223-9 5 Physical Examination Signs of Inspection and Medical Eponyms in Pericarditis Part I: 1761 to 1852.
- Clinical examination in cardiology, 2nd edition, B N Vijay Raghawa Rao.

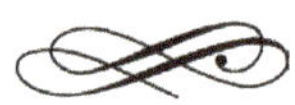

CHAPTER

6 Palpation of the Chest/Precordium

Palpation in CVS examination is probably the most important thing only next to auscultation.

Obviously, in palpation we try to confirm much of the findings that we got in inspection.

These points are discussed below.

Measuring the chest dimensions

→ We confirm the chest shape and take the AP and transverse diameters.

→ Normally the transverse diameter/AP diameter ratio is 7:5.

→ We place two cardboards, one in front of the chest and the other on the back with the patient in sitting posture. This distance gives us the AP diameter.

→ Similarly, by placing these two cardboards on both the sides of the chest (at the axilla level), we can measure the transverse diameter.

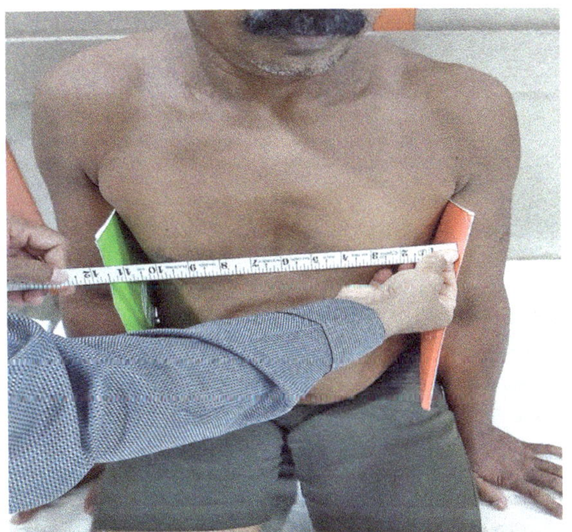

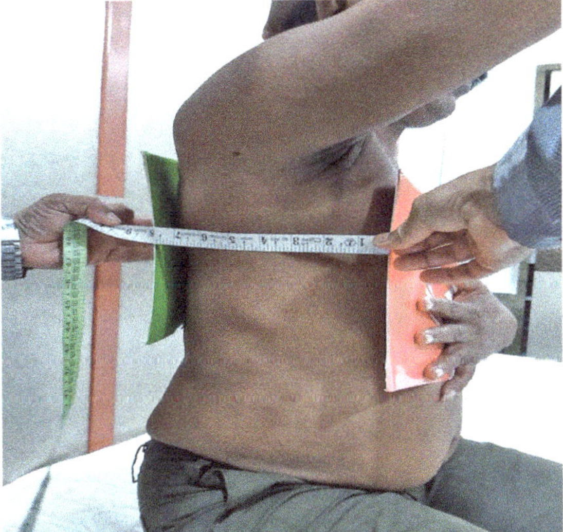

Fig. 6.1: Measuring the chest dimensions.

→ In the **barrel chest**, the **AP diameter > transverse diameter**.

Distended veins over the chest

→ The direction of blood flow in the veins can be judged by milking a section of the vein with two fingers to empty them and keeping the fingers firm there.

→ Releasing one finger at a time can reveal the direction of the flow.

→ If the **blood flows from above down**, it is **SVC obstruction**.

→ If the direction of flow is from **below to up**, it is **IVC obstruction**.

Tenderness of precordium

→ To rule out precordial tenderness is important because the patient may take it as a cardiac pain and may become anxious.

→ Many times during the winter season, the patient develops costochondritis (**Tietze syndrome**) and presents with symptoms of chest pain. On palpation, there is tenderness of the costochondral junction.

→ Similarly there could be chest tenderness in **acute pericarditis** and **myocarditis**.

Palpation of cardiac impulse, pulsations, sounds, thrills

→ Before we start the precordial palpation, do not forget the basics, i.e.; stand on the right side of the patient and rub both the hands together to warm them.

→ The trunk of the patient should be properly exposed till the waist.

→ The patient lies in a supine position with a slight upward inclination of 25^0-30^0. For cardiac apex, we make the patient lie in the left lateral position so that the apex is palpated better.

→ High frequency activities like S1, S2, opening snap should be felt with the proximal metacarpals and palm with firm pressure.

→ Low frequency activities like S3, S4 are felt with light pressure with the distal part of the fingers.

→ Thrills are felt just like the high frequency activities with firm pressure with the palm and distal fingers.

→ Also it is very important to time all the precordial pulsations with the carotid pulse (with the left hand) or by auscultation.

Palpation of the cardiac apex

→ As described in the section on inspection, location of the apical impulse is done in the sitting posture.

→ The palpation of the cardiac apex however, is first done in the 30^0-45^0 inclined supine position to confirm the site and then the patient is made to lie in the left lateral position (rotated around 90^0 from the supine position) to confirm the character/contour of the cardiac apex.

→ We should first palpate the apex with a flat palmar surface to locate it and then feel it with the ulnar border of the palm and finally pinpoint it with the right index finger for final localization and character.

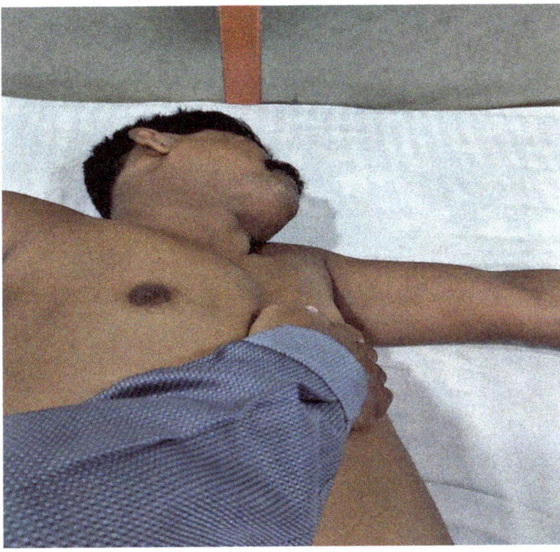

Fig. 6.2

→ The cardiac apex is palpated for its normal expected parameters like size, location, duration, character, and any other palpable sounds and thrills.

→ The cardiac apex is defined as the lateral most and lowest point of systolic outward motion felt on the chest wall in early systole followed by a very mild medial retraction in later part of the systole.

→ It is normally located at the 5th intercostal space in the midclavicular line or within 10 cm to the left of the midsternal line, occupying not > 2.5-3.0 cm in diameter, and lasts < 50% of the systole.

Abnormalities of the cardiac apex

→ Displaced cardiac apex, double/triple cardiac apex, diffuse cardiac apex, absent cardiac apex, etc is already discussed in detail in the section on Inspection of the anterior chest and precordium.

Cardiac apex contour/character

(1) **Sustained cardiac apex** and **hyperdynamic cardiac apex** has been already described in the previous section.

(2) **Tapping apex beat**

→ Seen in mitral stenosis (MS)

→ Due to the stenosis of the mitral valve, there is decreased LV filling which shortens the systolic thrust exerted by the LV on the chest wall (because of ejection of blood into the aorta). This gives the apex beat its sharp and tapping nature in MS.

→ This tapping apex beat is the palpable equivalent for the S1.

Low frequency sounds palpable at the cardiac apex

→ As mentioned earlier, low frequency activities are felt with light pressure with the distal part of the fingers.

→ These include S3, S4, pericardial knock (PK)

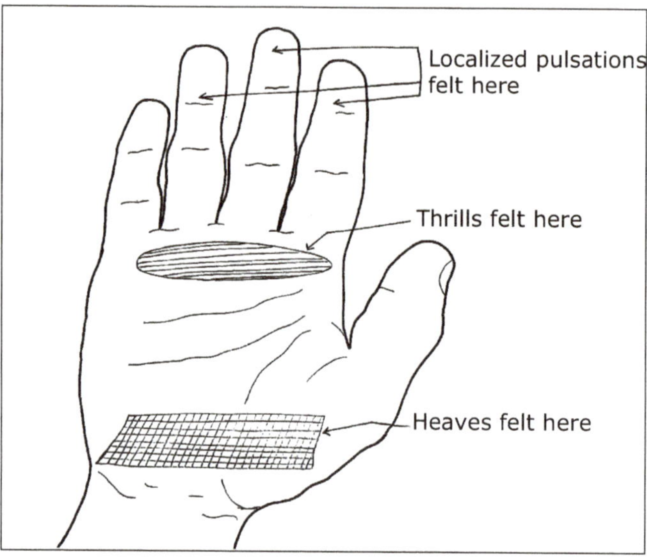

Fig. 6.3

→ It is indeed very uncommon to get these low frequency sounds palpable.

→ **S3**

- Also called protodiastolic sound or gallop
- Occurs at the end of rapid diastolic ventricular filling phase
- May be normal before age 40 years, but not after 40 years.
- Causes of palpable S3 are:

Ventricular dysfunction	Volume overload
(1) Cardiac failure	(1) Valvular regurgitation
(2) IHD	(2) Anemia
(3) DCM	(3) Pregnancy
(4) HCM	(4) AV fistula
(5) Valvular heart diseases like acute MR	(5) Hyperthyroidism
(6) Cor pulmonale	(6) Complete AV block
(7) Myocarditis	(7) Renal failure
	(8) Fluid overload

→ **S4**

- Occurs due to ↓ ventricular compliance leading to ↑ resistance to late diastolic ventricular filling due to atrial contraction (There is an increase in the LVEDP).
- Occurs just before S1, i.e; presystolic.
- Causes of palpable S4 are: LV hypertrophy states (AS,HCM), IHD, acute MR (due to enhanced filling of a non dilated ventricle), thyrotoxicosis and anemia (same mechanism as acute MR), physiologically in women above 40 years of age (rare).

→ **Pericardial knock**

- Indicates the termination of the rapid ventricular filling phase
- Occurs 0.06-0.08 seconds earlier than S3.
- Occurs in constrictive pericarditis.

High frequency sounds palpable at the cardiac apex

→ High frequency activities should be felt with the proximal metacarpals and palm with firm pressure.

→ These include loud S1, opening snap (OP), tumor plop, systolic ejection clicks.

→ **Loud S1**

- Indicates severe MS (leaflets are kept wide apart due to ↑ RAP and they close with great excursion producing loud S1).
- Can also be seen in states that cause a rapid rate of increase of the ventricular pressure like anemia, pregnancy, thyrotoxicosis etc.

→ **Tumor plop**

- Seen in atrial myxoma
- The mechanism is the same as that of loud S1.

→ **Opening snap**

- Occurs in MS due to sudden stoppage of thickened and pliable mitral valves during diastole with a raised LAP.
- Usually occurs 0.03-0.14 seconds after the S2.

→ **Ejection clicks**

- Also called ejection sounds.
- Occurs in pliable stenotic aortic valves, and nonstenotic bicuspid aortic valves.
- Ejection click best heard at the aortic area is caused by aortic root dilatation.

Thrills palpable at the cardiac apex

→ These are vibrations from the heart or the aorta which are transmitted to the chest wall and felt by the palpating hand.

→ Usually produced due to blood flowing through a stenotic lesion and producing Eddie currents that create vibrations.

→ Causes: MR (rare), VSD, MS.

→ Thrills synchronous with apical thrust (or carotid stroke) are systolic thrills.

→ Thrills asynchronous with apical thrust are diastolic thrills.

Friction rub palpable at the cardiac apex

→ Acute pericarditis

→ Best felt in the mid precordial region.

Palpation of the Left parasternal area (LPA)

→ LPA (roughly from the left 3rd to 6th ribs) pulsations and lifts are mainly due to abnormalities of the RV, mainly RV hypertrophy.

→ There could be LPA lifts or there could be RV palpable sounds like RV S3, RV S4.

LPA lift

→ LPA lifts are most commonly due to RV hypertrophy.

→ The LPA lift (sometimes heave) is palpated with the proximal part of the palm of the examiner, i.e.; the thenar and hypothenar area of the palm, with the fingers lifted up. The patient holds the breath in end expiration. Check for the movements of the hand.

→ Alternatively we can use the ulnar border of the right hand or three fingers of the right hand(index, middle and ring fingers) to palpate the 3rd, 4th, 5th intercostal spaces respectively to check for LPA lifts.

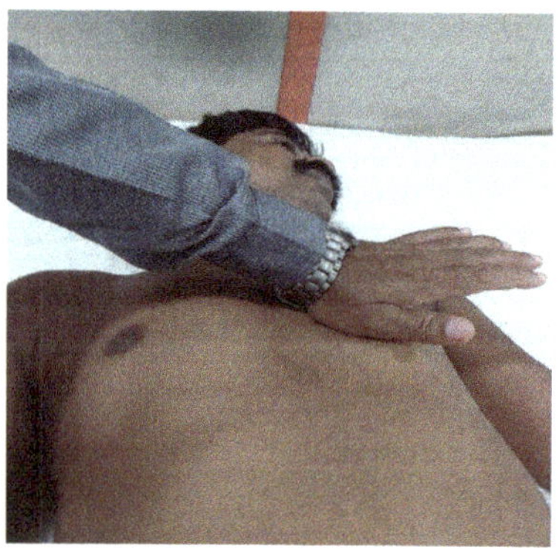
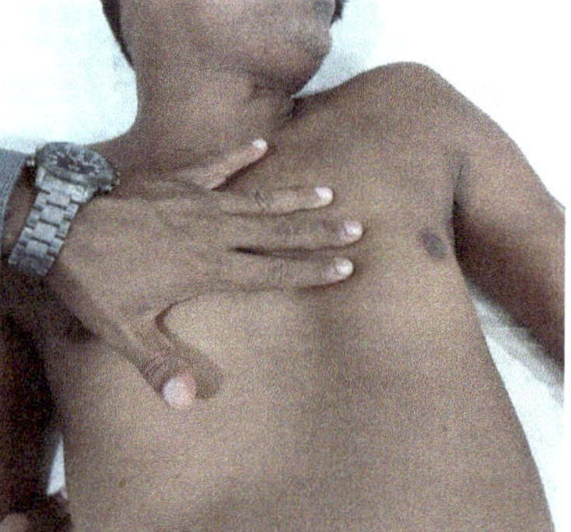
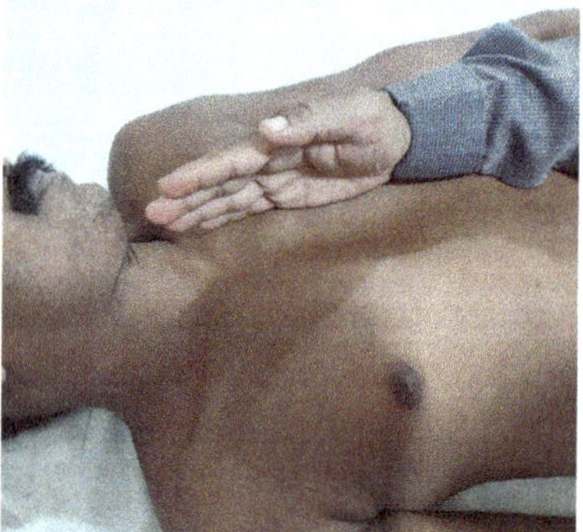

Fig. 6.4

→ A sustained LPA lift (heave) is seen in conditions causing RV hypertrophy with pulmonary hypertension like pulmonic stenosis (Grade 2/3), MS with PAH (Grade 2/3), cardiomyopathy, IPAH.

→ A hyperdynamic LPA lift indicates RV volume overload states like ASD (Grade 2/3) or TR (Grade 3/3). However, the development of PH in such conditions would change the lift to a sustained one.

→ LPA lift can also be seen with severe MR, in which the systolic expansion of the LA pushes the RV forward, producing the lift. However, the LPA lift produced by the LA expansion starts and terminates after the LV systolic beat.

→ Aneurysm of the LV that causes abnormal anterior movement during contraction can cause LPA lifts.

→ A mild PSA movement may be present normally in small children and thin individuals, which is a normal finding.

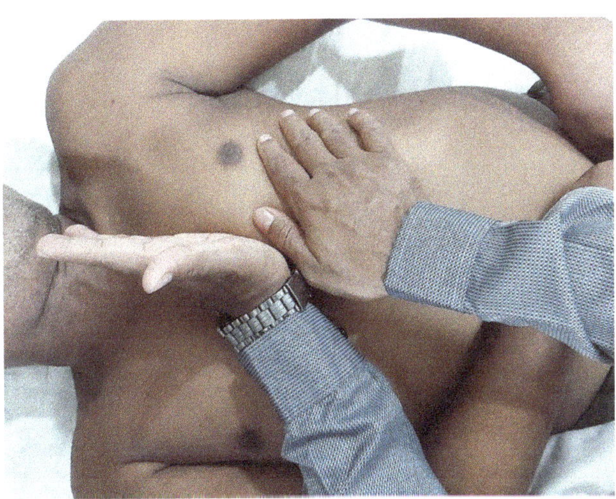

Fig. 6.5: Simultaneous palpation of the LPA lift and the cardiac apex.

Grades of LPA lift (AIIMS GRADING)

- Grade I - Can be seen but cannot be palpated
- Grade II - Can be seen, palpated and obliterated
- Grade III - Can be seen and palpated, but cannot be obliterated

RV S3

→ Although uncommon, RV S3 can be seen due to any cause leading to RV dysfunction

→ Also seen in volume overflow states like ASD, TR etc.

→ There is inspiratory augmentation of the RV S3.

RV S4

→ Classically associated with severe PS with PAH where the RV compliance is reduced.

Palpation of the tricuspid area (left lower sternum)

→ Opening snap of TS

→ Diastolic thrill of TS

→ Sometimes, diastolic rumble of severe TR

→ Systolic thrill of VSD

Palpation of the aortic area

→ High frequency sounds: Palpable A2 in aortic stenosis, hypertension, aortic root dilatation, TGA.

→ Systolic thrill of aortic stenosis (patient in sitting posture, leaning forward and respiration held in expiration).

→ Ejection sound of congenital aortic stenosis (may be better heard at the apex sometimes).

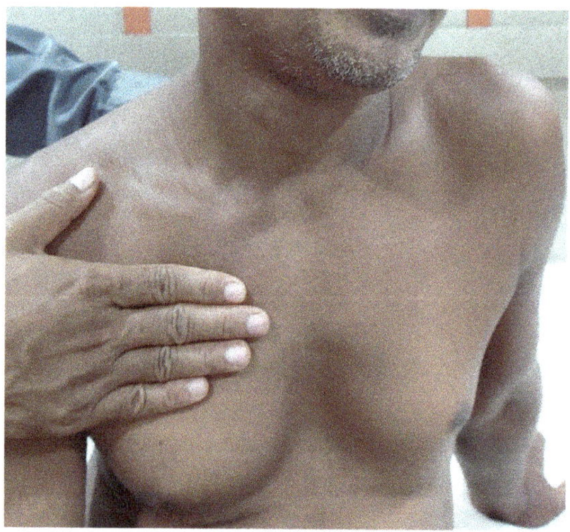

Fig. 6.6: Palpation of the aortic area.

Palpation on pulmonary area

→ High frequency sounds: Palpable P2 in PAH.

→ Ejection sound of PS.

→ Systolic thrill in PS (posture of the patient remains the same as in aortic area palpation).

→ Sometimes, early diastolic murmur of PR (Graham Steel murmur).

→ Continuous thrill: PDA (can also be below the left clavicle).

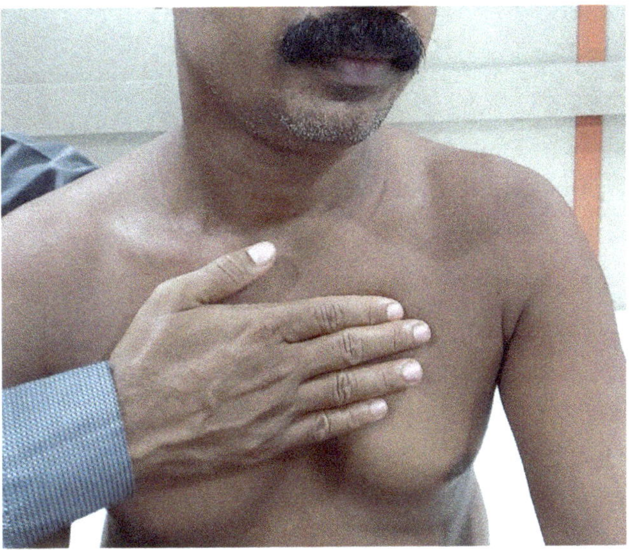

Fig. 6.7: Palpation of the pulmonary area.

Palpation of sub xiphoid area

→ Very specific for RV impulse.

→ Palpated with the hand over the epigastrium and the fingers facing the head of the patient

→ If the pulsations hit the fingertips then they are RV impulses. If the pulsations hit the palm then they are abdominal aortic pulsations. If the pulsations hit the lateral surface of the index finger then they are hepatic pulsations.

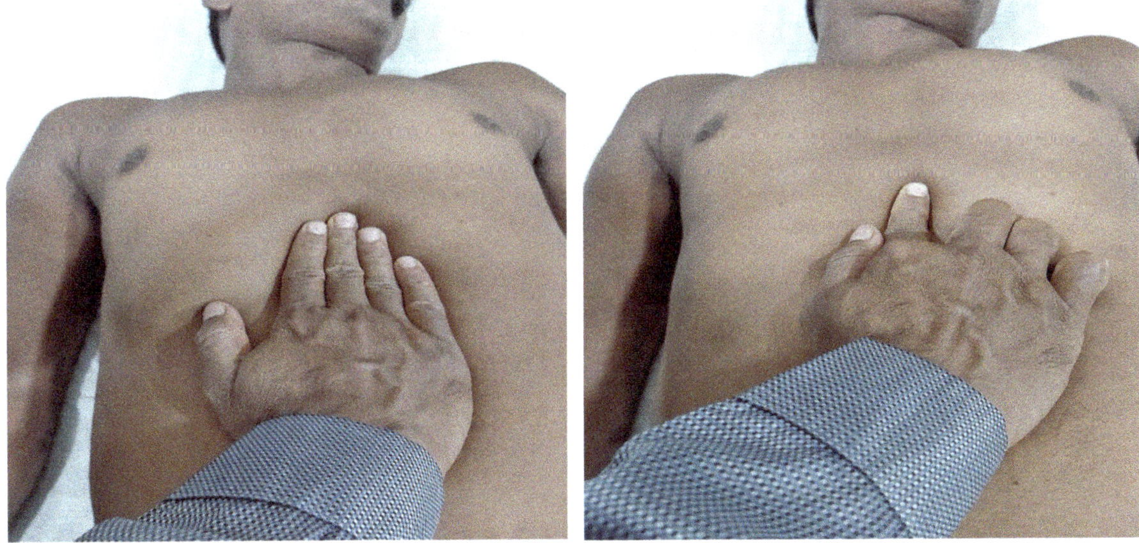

Fig. 6.8: Methods of palpation of the subxiphoid area.

Palpation of the right lower chest

→ Gives idea about RA enlargement in conditions like TR.

→ Impulse can be felt at the right 4th intercostal area also.

Tracheal Tug / Oliver's sign

→ This test is done to detect aortic arch aneurysm.

→ The patient sits with the neck extended. We apply upward pressure on the cricoid cartilage.

→ The presence of an arch of aorta aneurysm will exert a downward "tug" on the palpating fingers as the arch overlies the left main bronchus.

→ Abnormal pulsations from the large vessels of the neck will move the cricoid cartilage front and back, but not downwards as in aortic arch aneurysm.

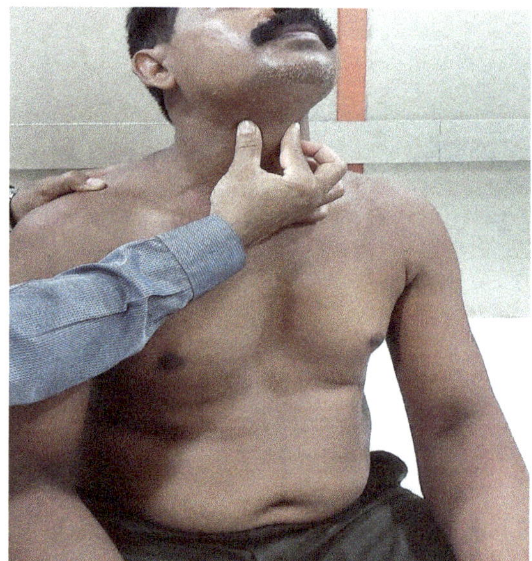

Fig. 6.9

Apex cardiogram

→ Recording of the low frequency precordial movements overlying the cardiac apex.

→ Uses:

- timing the cardiac events with a phonocardiogram
- mitral valve disease
- coronary artery disease

→ Movement of the precordium = cardiac movements + Changes in volume + pulsations of the great vessels.

→ Best places to record:

- Cardiac movement: apex
- Volume and consistency changes: parasternal area
- Pulsations of the great vessels: base of the heart

→ To record the apex cardiogram, the patient lies in a 45^0 propped up position. The apex beat is located in the lateral decubitus position and then a funnel is applied to the maximal impulse point which is connected to tubings which in turn connects to the piezo-electric recorder.

Normal apex cardiogram

→ Four phases:

- Phase 1: a wave
- Phase 2: systolic wave
- Phase 3: early ventricular filling wave(EFW)
- Phase 4: slow ventricular filling

→ Point O - lowest point between 2 and 3

→ Point F - indicates termination of early filling, between 3 and 4.

→ Matching the apex cardiogram components with the ECG waves:

- A wave starts with the apical part of the P wave in ECG
- Upstroke wave starts with the QRS complex
- Downstroke wave starts before the T wave finishes.

a wave (Phase 1) ⇒

→ Indicates atrial contraction phase (late ventricular filling)

→ Absent a wave: atrial fibrillation, MS

→ Increased size of a wave: AS, HTN, MR

Systolic wave (Phase 2) ⇒

→ Occurs due to ventricular contraction

→ Has several components like upstroke, plateau, downstroke etc.

→ O point is the lowest point of the downstroke where there is opening of the A-V valves and filling of the ventricles occur. This point may indicate an opening snap in MS.

Phase 3 ⇒

→ Starts with point O and terminates at point F

→ Indicates the rapid filling phase

→ Diminished in MS

→ Sharp and prominent in MR, due to increased atrial blood during rapid filling.

→ Point F indicates the end of rapid filling and coincides with the S3 in MR.

Phase 4 ⇒

→ Indicates late phase of ventricular filling and terminates with the next a wave

→ Phase 3 and Phase 4 cannot be distinguished in severe MS.

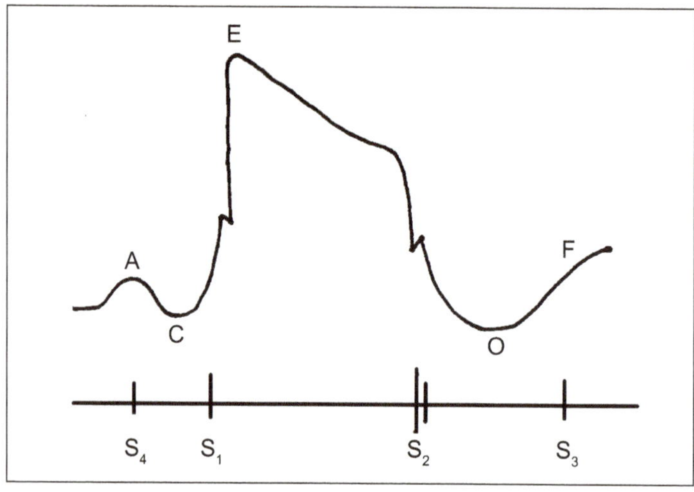

Fig. 6.10

References

- Constrictive Pericarditis ANURAG MEHTA, M.D., MAHAVEER mHTA, M.D., ABNASH c. JAN, M.D; Clin. Cardiol. 22, 334-344 (1999).
- A textbook of symptoms and physical signs, 13th edition, Rustom Jal Vakil and Aspi F. Golwalla.
- Clinical examination in cardiology, 2nd edition by B N VIJAY RAGHAWA RAO.
- Clinical methods in cardiology by B SOMA RAJU.
- Clinical Methods: The History, Physical, and Laboratory Examinations. 3rd edition. Chapter 25 The Fourth Heart Sound; Eric S. Williams.; Chapter 24 The Third Heart Sound, Mark E. Silverman; Chapter 22The First Heart Sound Joel M. Felner; Chapter 28 Ejection Clicks William R. Jacobs.
- Circulation, Volume XXII, September 1960; Clinical Recognition of Tricuspid Stenosis By JOSEPH K. PERLOFF, M.D., AND WV. PROCTOR HARVEY, M.D.
- Chest journal, The Value of the Apex Cardiogram in Coronary Artery Disease.
- A. Benchimol, M.D., Peter Maroko, M.D. October 1968 Volume 54, Issue 4, Pages 378-380.
- Brit. Heart J., 1963 25, 697. The apex cardiogram: Its normal features explained by those found in heart disease by N. Coulshed and E. J. Epstein

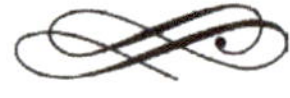

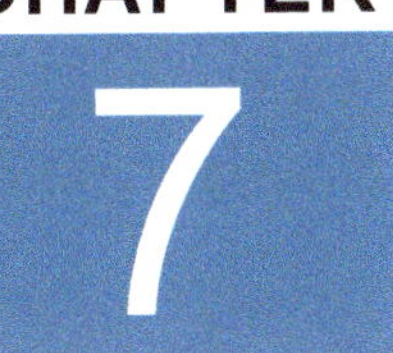

CHAPTER 7 Percussion of the CVS

Percussion was introduced by Joseph L Auenbrugger as a new tool in clinical examination.

In percussion we interpret the sounds produced by stroking the chest/precordium with our fingers(pitch, character, intensity) and also feel the resistance obtained.

Two methods of percussion

→ **Direct method** ⇨ where we stroke the chest wall directly by the fingers.

→ **Indirect method** ⇨ where we place our left middle finger on the chest wall and indirectly strike the chest by striking on the left hand finger with our right middle finger. The left middle finger absorbing the strike is called Pleximeter and the right middle finger giving the strike is called Plexor. Bony prominences like the clavicle can be directly percussed.

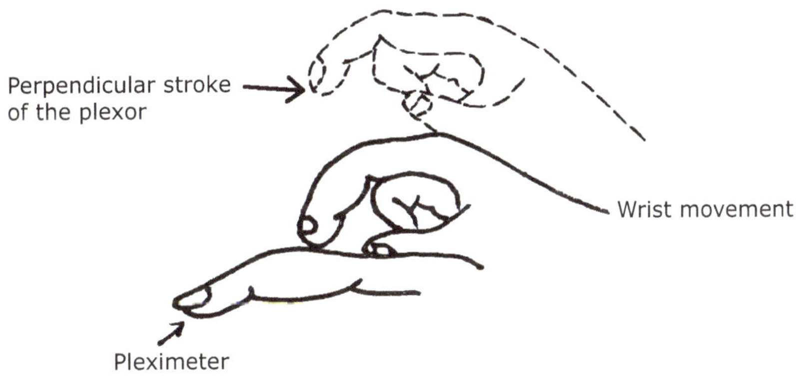

Fig. 7.1: Indirect method of percussion.

Some rules of percussion of the chest wall for CVS

→ We know that lungs overlie most of the heart in the thoracic cavity. Percussion over the lungs would give a resonant note.

→ Hence, when we percuss, we should start from outside, i.e.; from the lateral chest and move towards the heart (centripetally).

→ This is going to give us a resonant note of the lungs initially which changes to a dull note as we approach the heart. The change of note from resonant to dull is easy to perceive rather than the reverse.

→ Commonly it is a practice to keep the pleximeter parallel to the ribs and intercostal space (ICS). But some people may prefer to keep it parallel to the cardiac border (perpendicular to the ribs).

Cardiac percussion proper

→ The purpose of percussing the CVS is to mark the left and right cardiac borders.

→ For the left cardiac border, we locate the apex beat at the 5th ICS and start percussing from the axilla towards the heart. As we reach the cardiac border, there is a slight dullness of the note. This area nearly lies at or just lateral to the apex beat itself.

→ similar percussion is done at the left 4th and 3rd ICS.

→ Normally the midsternal to cardiac border distance is around 7 - 9 cm in 5th ICS and 3 - 3.5 cm in 3rd ICS.

→ An increase in the 5th ICS cardiac border distance is seen in pericardial effusion, left heart enlargement, a right sided pleural effusion pushing the heart to the left, etc.

→ An increased 3rd ICS cardiac border distance may be seen in enlargement of the left atrial appendage or dilatation of the pulmonary artery.

→ For the right cardiac border, we first mark the liver dullness by percussing from above in the midclavicular line on the right side. Usually the upper border of liver dullness is in the 5th ICS.

→ Once this is done, we start percussing for the right cardiac border from the 4th ICS to above.

→ Usually the right cardiac border is retrosternal.

→ If the midsternal to right cardiac border distance exceeds 1 cm, it may indicate RA enlargement or pericardial effusion.

Percussion of the aortic and pulmonary areas

→ Ideally there should be a resonant note.

→ A dull note indicates pathology.

→ Dull aortic area percussion : aneurysm of aorta, tumor of the mediastinum, etc.

→ Dull pulmonary area percussion : dilatation of pulmonary artery, PDA, etc.

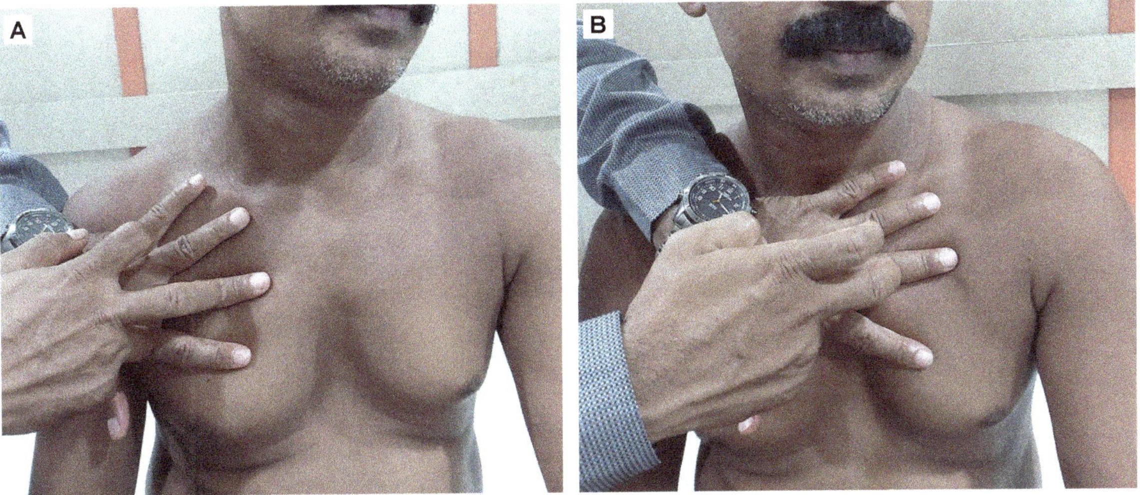

Fig. 7.2: (A) Percussion of the aortic area; (B) Percussion of the pulmonary area.

> **NOTE**
>
> At the end, it is important to detect situs solitus by percussion of the stomach fundus on the left and liver dullness on the right.

References

- A textbook of symptoms and physical signs,13th edition, Rustom Jal Vakil and Aspi F.Golwalla.
- Clinical examination in cardiology, 2nd edition, B N VIJAY RAGHAWA RAO.

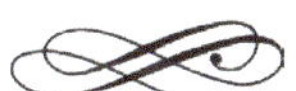

CHAPTER

8 Auscultation of the CVS

The word "**Auscultation**" was coined by Laennec and is derived from the Latin word "**auscultare**" which means "**to listen carefully**".

Cardiac auscultation is a more than 200 years old clinical art that helps clinicians to learn the disease and decide whether or not to subject the patient to other higher investigations.

It is from the era of Hippocrates that the art of auscultation has been practised. They used to put their ears directly on the patient's chest wall to listen for the pulmonary sounds, a technique called "immediate auscultation".

However, it would look awkward to put the ears on a female patient's chest to listen to her heart beats. This led Laennec to make a paper tube and place it on the chest of the patient to hear the heart beats followed by a hollow wooden tube used for the same. And finally in 1826, Laennec succeeded to invent the Stethoscope which proved to be a blessing for the art of auscultation.

When talking about cardiac sounds, **pitch** relates to the **frequency** of the sound or murmur.

Low frequency heart sounds:

→ 25 - 150 Hz

→ Pitch - low

→ S3, S4, Mid diastolic murmur (MDM) in MS or TS, Pericardial knock(PK), Austin Flint murmur, etc.

High frequency heart sounds:

→ > 300 Hz

→ Pitch - high

→ S2, Systolic murmur of MR, Diastolic murmur of AR, OS, Ejection clicks, etc.

Mixed frequency heart sounds:

→ S1, Murmur of AS, VSD, PS, etc.

Most of the cardiac sound frequencies range between 30-80 Hz and the human ear can detect frequencies between 16000-18000 HZ. However, the optimal human auditory acuity ranges between 1000-2000 Hz.

It is for this reason why we use a stethoscope to hear cardiac sounds.

Also, human ears can differentiate two sounds as "distinct" only if both the sounds are separated by a time interval not < 0.02 seconds.

Factors that hampers cardiac sound auscultation quality

→ Thick chest, excess breast tissue, muscular chest, COPD, pleural effusion, pericardial effusion.

→ Excess noise in the examination room. Ideally the sound level in the examination room should be < 35 db. Mainly affects the high frequency sounds.

→ Age factor also plays a vital role as there could be presbycusis wherein the higher frequency sounds can be easily missed during auscultation.

Know your Stethoscope

Stethoscope is still an important bedside instrument for all physicians as it gives immense information about the disease process if used logically and correctly.

A stethoscope consists of a dual chest piece with a valve that helps to switch the bell and diaphragm as and when required, the tubing, binaural connector, and the earpieces.

A good stethoscope is one that does not distort the sound and gives valid information about the sound quality, characteristics, frequency, etc.

Bell of stethoscope

→ Should be trumpet shaped

→ Minimum diameter should be 1 inch

→ Should have a rubber rim that ensures a proper skin contact, prevents air leak, helps increase the diameter and doesn't get cold in winter months.

→ Bell detects the low frequency sounds when applied very lightly to the skin surface. It should not be pressed firmly to the skin, else it acts as the diaphragm and amplifies the high frequency sounds and blocks the low frequency ones.

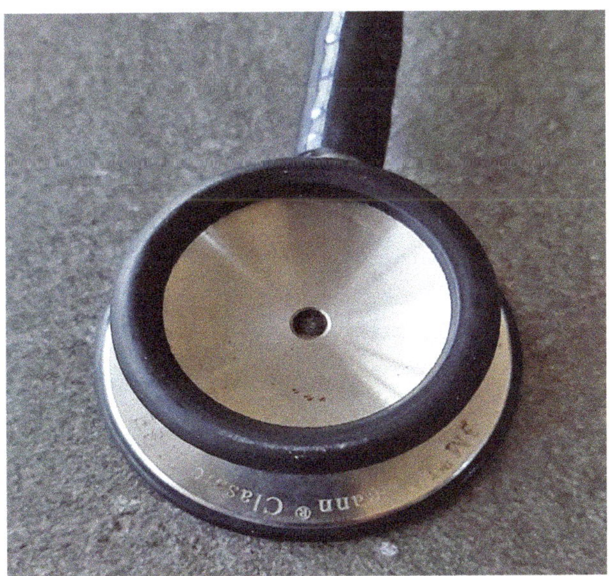

Fig. 8.1

Diaphragm of stethoscope

→ It is the high frequency detecting component of the chest piece.

→ Should be applied with firm pressure which blocks the low frequency sounds and transmits the high frequency ones.

→ It should have a diameter of at least 1.5 inch.

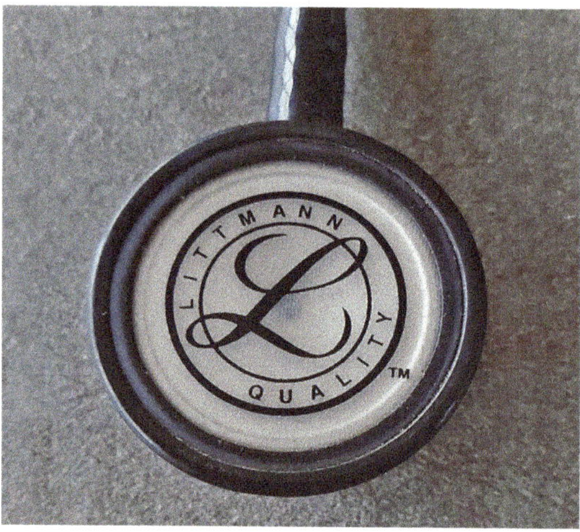

Fig. 8.2

Tube of stethoscope

→ Ideal length should be 10-15 inches and ideal internal diameter 3 mm.

→ Double lumen tubing with an external single tube is ideal.

→ Should be thick, and made of plastic to block external noise and avoid tube buckling.

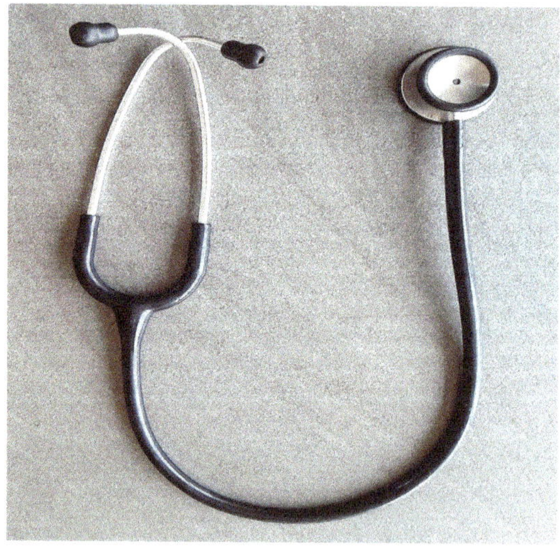

Fig. 8.3

Binaurals and earpiece

→ Binaurals should be oriented slightly anteriorly similar to the direction of the ear canal.

→ Earpiece should not be too small as it can go deep inside the ear canal and may cause occlusion.

→ Earpiece should be soft and non traumatic.

→ Larger earpieces are better.

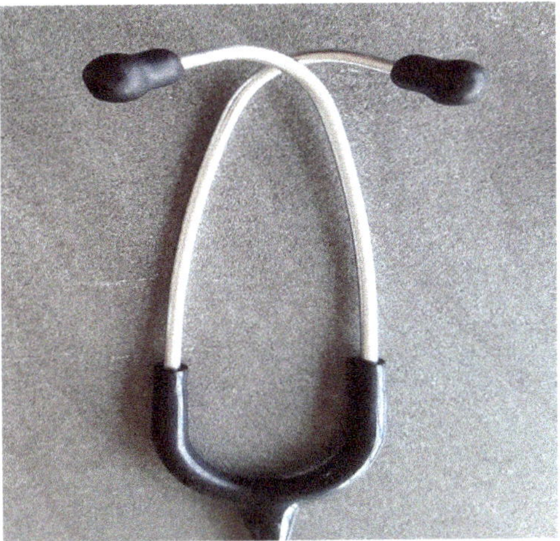

Fig. 8.4

Proper care and cleaning of the stethoscope

→ The stethoscope is a delicate instrument. If we drop it down frequently or if the diaphragm/bell is hit accidently then the quality of sound transmission may hamper.

→ Folding the tubings and keeping the stethoscope in the pockets of the apron daily may damage the instrument. Better is to keep the stethoscope hanging around the neck during the clinical rounds.

→ The ear pieces should be regularly checked for any crack or wax accumulation.

→ Tubing leaks can be checked by blowing through one ear piece and blocking the other.

→ Cleaning the stethoscope is very very important which the majority of us forget to do. It can cause cross infections among patients and can also infect us and our family members.

→ Proper cleaning can decrease the infection rate from 84% to 33% as per a research, especially MRSA induced infections.

→ The stethoscope can be cleaned with ethyl or isopropyl alcohol based sanitizers that physicians use.

→ It is recommended to clean the diaphragm and bell first and then sanitize our hands before the rounds so that by the time we finish our hand sanitization, the stethoscope has already dried up and is ready for use.

Areas of auscultation

Before proceeding for auscultation, it is very important to know the proper history of the patient's illness, do a good general examination, inspection, palpation and percussion of the CVS so that it forms a proper framework for the auscultation and helps us arrive at the most probable clinical diagnosis.

The examination room should be quiet, well illuminated, and should not be too hot or too cold.

The patient's trunk is exposed properly upto the waist and we stand on the right side of the patient.

The areas of cardiac auscultation are:

→ **Mitral area:** at the cardiac apex

→ **Aortic area:** right 2nd ICS

→ **Pulmonary area:** left 2nd ICS

→ **Tricuspid area:** 4th and 5th ICS near the left of the sternum

→ **Erb's area:** left 3rd ICS. Also called the Neoaortic area.

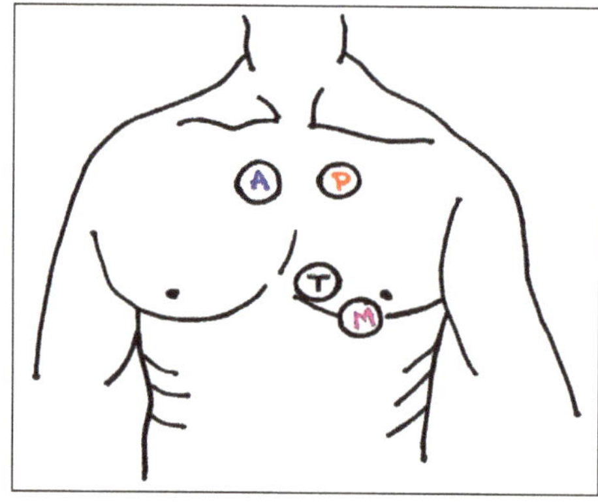

Fig. 8.5

The auscultation should not be restricted only to these above mentioned areas as there are many other areas where one can get abnormal heart sounds and murmurs.

These areas are:

→ **Axilla:** Pansystolic murmur (PSM) of MR radiates to the axilla when tha anterior mitral leaflet (AML) is involved.

→ **Interscapular area:** for the murmurs of coarctation of aorta and descending aortic aneurysm.

→ **Right chest:** to rule out dextrocardia.

→ **Carotids:** aortic SM are conducted to the carotids.

→ **Left infraclavicular area:** for the continuous murmur of PDA.

→ **Epigastrium:** murmur of TR

→ **Peripheral arteries:** especially femorals bilaterally, for Duroziez murmur in AR.

The technique of auscultation

While we start auscultation, it is very important that we are aware of the phases of the cardiac cycle that we are listening to, i.e; systole and diastole.

S1 reflects the onset of systole and S2 reflects the onset of diastole.

Simultaneous with the auscultation, we palpate the carotid pulse or the apex beat.

S1 is followed immediately by the carotid upstroke and the beginning of the outward thrust of the apex beat. S2 occurs slightly later.

The "inching" technique of Levine and Harvey

This is a method of systematic auscultation wherein, we start the auscultation at the mitral area (apex) and keep moving slowly to the axilla, from there to the tricuspid area along the left lower sternum, to the neoaortic area along the sternum and then to the pulmonary, aortic and clavicular areas and finally auscultate the carotids.

By this method, we set a chain of auscultation of all the cardiac areas without missing any.

The technique of "selective listening"

This technique was developed by **Dr. W. Proctor Harvey.**

This technique is the **HEART** of a proper cardiac auscultation.

This method is based on the principle of concentrating on one phase of the cardiac cycle at a time in terms of either cardiac sounds or murmurs.

We use the bell and diaphragm both, at every cardiac area and divide systole and diastole into three parts- early, mid, and late.

Also we focus on only one segment of the cardiac cycle at a time, e.g.; when we want to assess the systole, we focus on the S1 in early, mid or late systole.

Cardiac sounds are attended first followed by cardiac murmurs.

With this technique, there is very little chance of missing any abnormal cardiac sound.

However, we should not forget that abnormal cardiac sounds are heard only when we look for them with proper auscultatory techniques and sheer concentration and obviously when our basic knowledge about cardiology is clear.

The time taken for each auscultation may decrease once we start gaining experience and auscultate more and more patients. We may even close our eyes during the auscultation for better concentration.

Positions for auscultation

(1) Mitral area ⇨ Left lateral decubitus

(2) Tricuspid area ⇨ Supine

(3) Basal areas ⇨ Sitting and leaning forward

(4) Tricuspid murmur ⇨ Right lateral decubitus

Apart from the above mentioned procedures of auscultation, the patient should also be auscultated in the standing and supine positions and subjected to additional maneuvers like respiration, isometric exercises, passive leg raising, Valsalva and Muller maneuvers and inhalation of amyl nitrate, that causes changes in the pre- and afterloads and make the cardiac sounds and murmurs more prominent.

These techniques are called Dynamic auscultation.

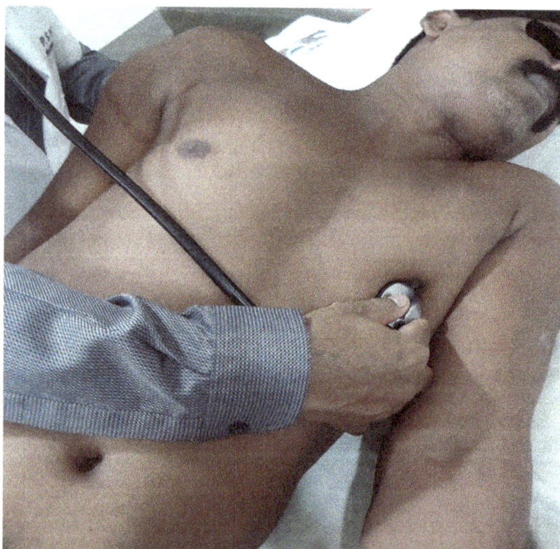

Fig. 8.6: Auscultation of the mitral area in left lateral decubitus position.

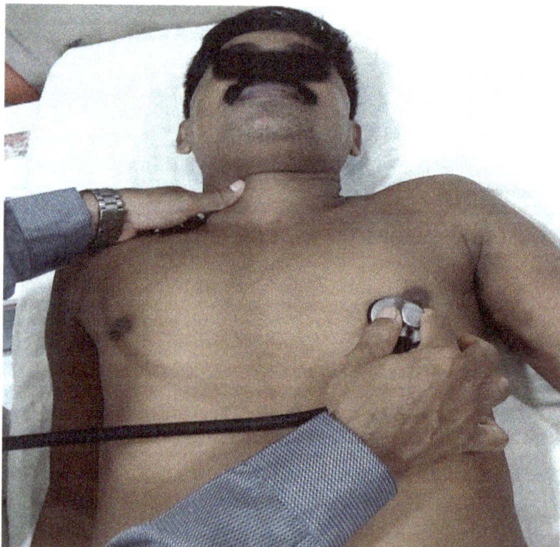

Fig. 8.7: Simultaneous auscultation of the mitral area and palpation of the carotid pulse.

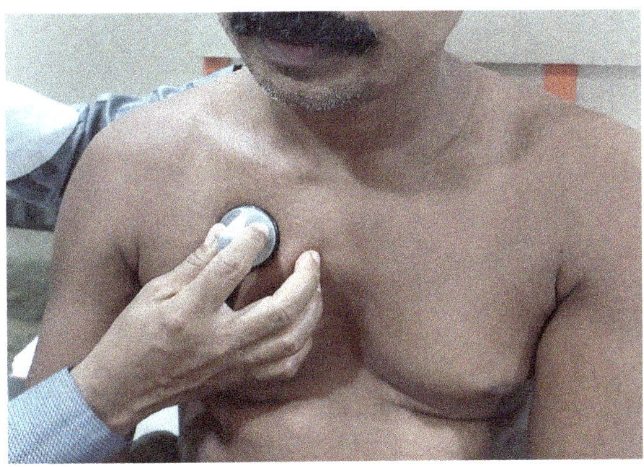

Fig. 8.8: Auscultation of the aortic area.

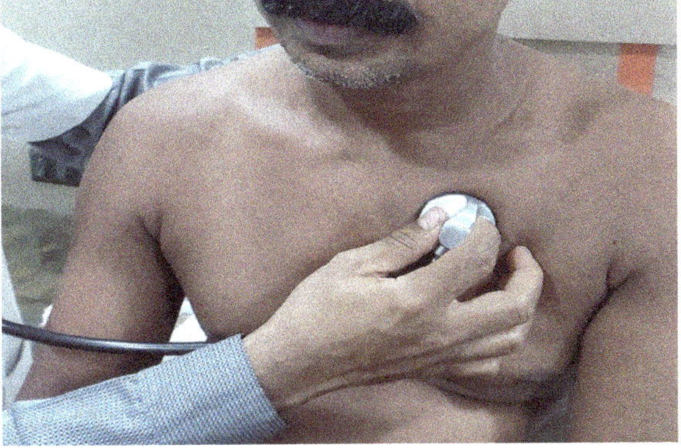

Fig. 8.9: Auscultation of the pulmonary area.

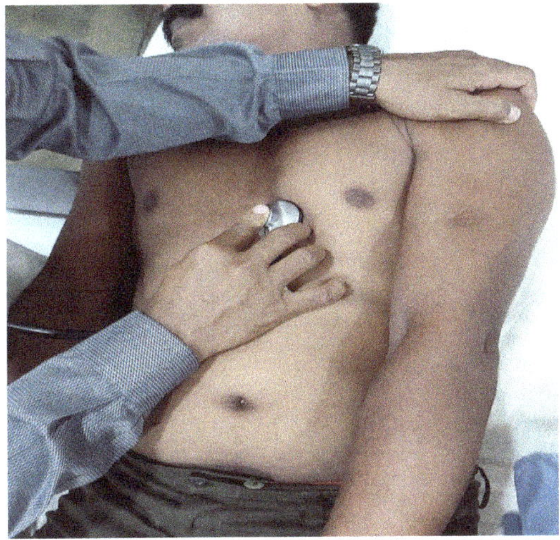

Fig. 8.10: Auscultation of the tricuspid area in right lateral tilt position.

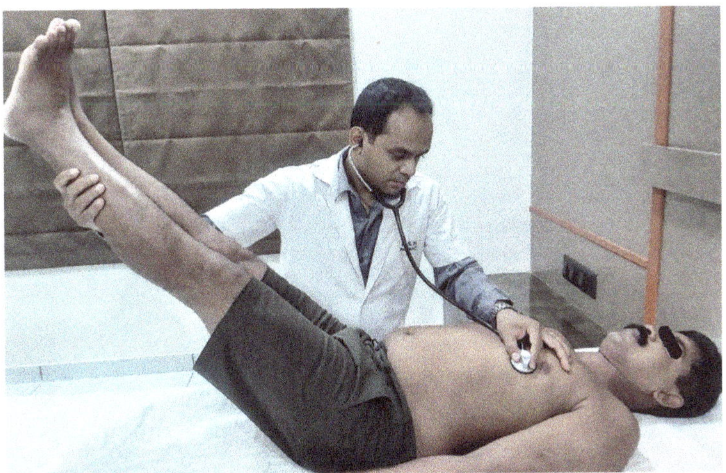

Fig. 8.11: Auscultation with passive leg raising.

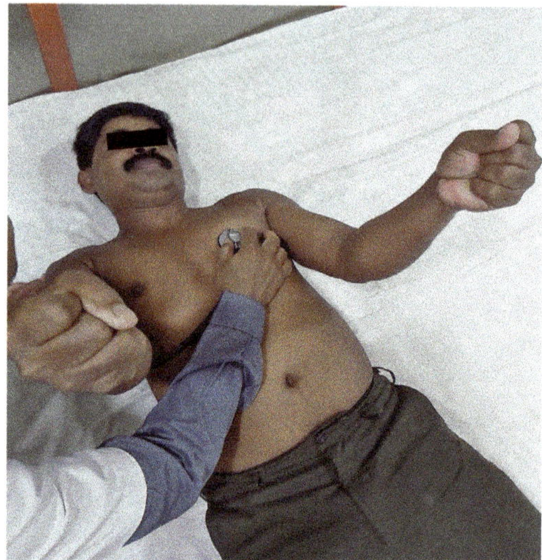

Fig. 8.12: Auscultation with sustained hand grip.

Heart sounds

Heart sounds are produced due to sudden stoppage of blood within the CVS that initiates vibration in the valves and adjacent heart walls and major vessels around the heart. Every heart sound has its own characteristic intensity, frequency (pitch), and timber.

Classification of heart sounds

Depending on frequency (discussed earlier)

(1) Low frequency ⇨ S3, S4, Pericardial knock (PK)

(2) High frequency ⇨ S2, OS, ejection clicks, non ejection sounds, tumor plops, pericardial rub.

(3) Medium frequency ⇨ S1

Depending on the phases of the cardiac cycle

(1) Systolic:

Early systolic ⇨ Ejection sounds (aortic and pulmonary), prosthetic valves closure sound

Mid/late systolic ⇨ Non ejection clicks

(2) Diastolic:

Early diastolic ⇨ Prosthetic valves opening sound, OS, PK, tumor plops

Mid diastolic ⇨ S3

Late diastolic ⇨ S4

References

- Journal of Multidisciplinary Healthcare 2019:12 183–189; The first 200 years of cardiac auscultation. and future perspectives by Maria Rosa Montinari and Sergio Minelli.
- Synopsis of cardiac physical diagnosis; 2nd edition; Jonathan Abrams.
- Clinical examination in cardiology; 2nd edition; B N VIJAY RAGHAWA RAO.
- The art and science of cardiac physical examination; 2nd edition; Narasimhan Ranganathan.

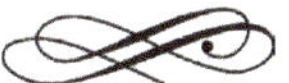

CHAPTER 9 The First Heart Sound (S1)

The first heart sound or S1 reflects the beginning of ventricular systole and occurs due to closure of the mitral and tricuspid valves (M1 and T1 components). The mitral valve closes just before the tricuspid valve.

However, apart from this valve closure sound, the S1 also has some inaudible vibrations as its components. These vibrations are the LV muscle contraction vibrations and the vascular vibrations that occur as the blood is pushed into the aorta and pulmonary artery as the LV contracts.

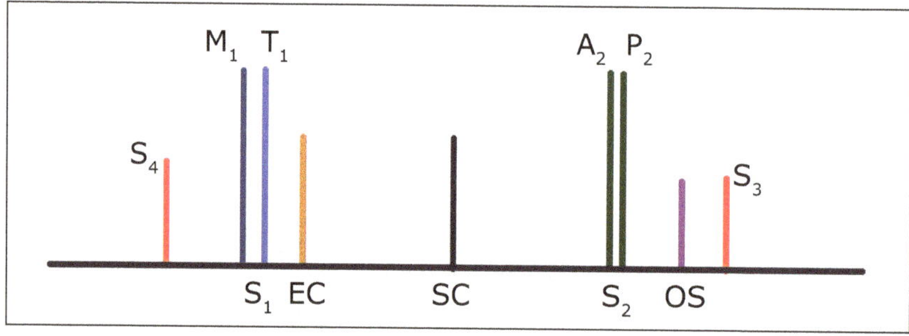

Fig. 9.1: The heart sounds.

Normal characteristics of S1

Frequency: Medium

Auscultation with stethoscope: Using the diaphragm

Best heard at: Apex

Timing: Matching with the carotid pulse or the apex beat

Duration: 0.14 second (S2 is shorter than S1 due to more taut semilunar valves than the AV valves, hence they vibrate for a lesser duration)

Time of separation between M1 and T1: 0.02-0.03 sec, hence perceived as a single S1

Clinical aspects of S1

→ Best heard at the apex.

→ Low pitched and longer than S2.

→ If S1 ≥ S2 at the base, the S1 is said to be loud or accentuated.

→ T1 best heard at the left lower border of sternum

→ Splitting of S1 also best heard at the left lower border of sternum. This split can be normal in upto 40% individuals.

NOTE

S2 has a higher frequency than S1 because:

⇨ Semilunar valves are more taut than AV valves

⇨ Elastic coefficient of the arterial walls > ventricular chambers.

Factors determining the Intensity of S1

(1) Structural normalcy of the mitral valve (MV) apparatus:

⇨ Mitral valve apparatus consists of the leaflets, papillary muscles, chordae tendineae, annulus, LV muscle.

⇨ If any of the mitral valve apparatus components is damaged structurally, it may lead to a defect in the intensity of S1. Normal mitral leaflets: Thin + pliable.

⇨ Severe MR → improper approximation of the leaflets → ↓ S1

⇨ IE → damaged leaflet tissue → ↓ S1

⇨ Very severe MS with severe valve calcification → ↓ S1

(2) PR interval:

⇨ The normal PR interval is 120-200 msec.

⇨ When the PR interval is short around 80-120 msec, the LV pressure is high while the LV-LA pressure crossover takes place which closes the widely separated MV with great force leading to ↑ S1, e.g.; WPW syndrome, Lown-Ganong-Levine syndrome.

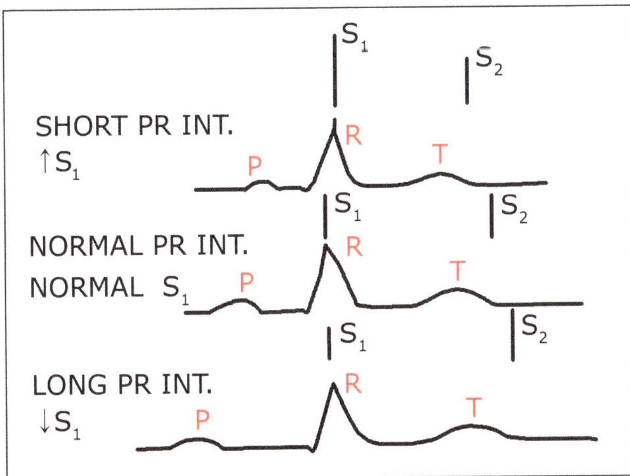

Fig. 9.2

- ⇨ When the PR is normal, we get a normal S1.
- ⇨ When the PR interval is > 200 msec, the MV closes before the LV pressure could rise, leading to a ↓ S1. (Other causes of premature MV closure are Acute severe AR, AR with LV dysfunction).

(3) Integrity of the isovolumetric contraction phase:

- ⇨ During isovolumetric contraction, the LV contracts as a closed chamber and there is a steep rate of rise of pressure, i.e.; dp/dt that closes the MV leaflets. Hence, any condition that affects this phase causes a ↓ S1.
- ⇨ **Severe MR, LV aneurysm** → abnormal isovolumetric contraction → reduced dp/dt → slow valve closure → ↓ S1.
- ⇨ **Severe AR** → poor isovolumetric contraction with ↑ LVEDP leading to premature closure of the MV → ↓ S1.
- ⇨ **VSD** may cause a ↓ S1 due to abnormal isovolumetric contraction but, very often both the ventricles act as a single chamber and lead to a normal S1.

(4) Proper myocardial contraction:

- ⇨ Conditions causing increased myocardial contraction will lead to an ↑ **S1** due to ↑ dp/dt, e.g.; **hypoglycemia, exercise, hyperthyroidism, ASD (↑ flow across the TV), beta2 agonists, hyperdynamic states**, etc.
- ⇨ Poor myocardial contraction will cause a ↓ S1 due to ↓ dp/dt leading to a reduced velocity of valve closure, e.g.; **IHD, cardiomyopathies, beta blockers, verapamil**, **LBBB** (also leads to premature MV closure), etc.

(5) Heart rate:

- ⇨ Tachycardia → ↓ PR and ↑ contractility (Treppe phenomenon) → valve wide open → ↑ S1.
- ⇨ Bradycardia has the opposite role.

(6) Thoracic abnormalities and other factors:

- ⇨ Thick chest wall, large breasts, COPD, pleural effusion, pericardial effusion → ↓ S1.
- ⇨ Lean individual → ↑ S1.

NOTE

In mitral stenosis (MS), there is an ↑ S1 because there is a presystolic gradient between the LA and LV which keeps the valve leaflets wide apart just prior to the onset of systole. With the onset of systole, there is an ↑ dp/dt which closes the widely separated valve leaflets with great velocity causing the ↑ S1. However, in MS the valves should be mobile and thick, else a severely calcified MS may lead to an absent S1 also.

LA myxoma and TS leads to an ↑ S1 due to the similar mechanism as MS.

Table 9.1

LOUD S1	SOFT S1
Mitral stenosis	Severely calcified MS
LA myxoma	Severe AR
Tricuspid stenosis	Severe MR
Exercise	IHD
Hyperdynamic states	Cardiomyopathy
ASD	LBBB
WPW syndrome	Ventricular aneurysm
Lown-Ganong-Levine syndrome	Myocarditis

Variable intensity of S1:

⇨ Occurs when there is no fixed PR interval

⇨ Atrial fibrillation, CHB with AV dissociation, varying block in AT, VTach+AV dissociation, second degree AV block, etc.

Splitting of the S1

S1 is said to be split when M1 and T1 are separated by a time interval of > 0.03 seconds.

This split can be best appreciated at the left lower sternal border with the diaphragm of a stethoscope.

Widely split S1 (due to delayed T1): RBBB, LV pacing, Ebstein anomaly, TS, RA myxoma, etc.

Reverse splitting of S1 (due to delayed M1): MS, RV pacing, Rv ectopics, LA myxoma, etc.

Pulmonary and aortic clicks creating false perception of a split S1

(1) Many times, a loud pulmonary ejection click may be perceived as a component of S1 and it may be taken as a split S1.

However, pulmonary ejection clicks are best heard at the left 2nd ICS and they would decrease with deep inspiration.

(2) An aortic click may sometimes give a false split S1 type picture.

On making the patient stand, there is ↓ venous return that in turn causes ↓ LA and LVED pressures and a ↓dp/dt ratio which widens the split and helps detect the false S1 split.

References

- Synopsis of cardiac physical diagnosis; 2nd edition; Jonathan Abrams.
- Clinical examination in cardiology; 2nd edition; B N VIJAY RAGHAWA RAO.
- The art and science of cardiac physical examination; 2nd edition; Narasimhan Ranganathan.
- Clinical Methods: The History, Physical, and Laboratory Examinations. 3rd edition. Chapter 22 The First Heart Sound by JOEL M. FELNER.

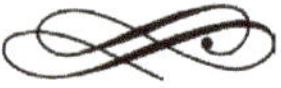

CHAPTER

10 The Second Heart Sound (S2)

The second heart sound (S2) indicates the end of ventricular systole and the beginning of the diastole.

It occurs due to the closure of the semilunar valves and the vibrations generated due to sudden deceleration of the blood in the aorta and pulmonary artery, as they hit the closed leaflets retrogradely.

The aortic component (A2) occurs earlier than the pulmonary component (P2) and is louder too. This property of A2 is due to a higher pressure and shorter hangout interval of the aorta.

Normal characteristics of S2

Frequency: High

Auscultation with stethoscope: Using the diaphragm

Best heard at: A2 - aortic area (and also at pulmonary area and apex), P2 - pulmonary area.

Duration: 0.11 second (S2 is shorter than S1 due to more taut semilunar valves than the AV valves, hence they vibrate for a lesser duration).

Time of separation between A2 and P2:

With inspiration ⇨ 0.04-0.05 seconds

With expiration ⇨ < 0.03 seconds (if > 0.04 seconds, the S2 is said to be split)

A2 louder than P2: Because of the higher aortic pressure

A2 occurring earlier than P2: Because of a shorter aortic hangout interval.

The concept of "Hangout interval"

With the end of the ventricular systole, we expect the semilunar valves to close as the ventricular pressure falls below the arterial pressures.

However, this doesn't happen and the semilunar valves close slightly later than this pressure crossover time.

This time lag is known as the hangout interval.

The hangout interval depends upon:

→ arterial pressures

→ arterial distensibility

→ elastic recoil

→ respiratory phase

The aortic hangout interval < pulmonary hangout interval due to more pressure in aorta and less compliance.

Normal split S2

- With inspiration, the pulmonary vascular impedance is reduced that increases the hangout interval, prolonging the pulmonary valve closure time leading to splitting of the A2-P2.

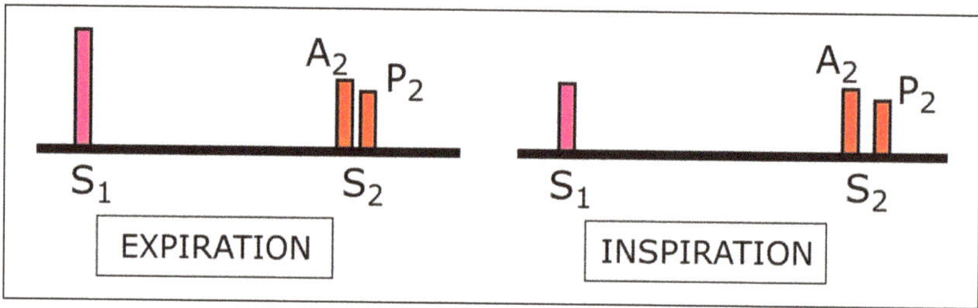

Fig. 10.1

To explain this in a better way

(1) Inspiration ⇨ ↓intrathoracic pressure ⇨ ↑RV venous return ⇨ ↑RV ejection time ⇨ ↑ hangout interval ⇨ delayed pulmonary valve closure ⇨ delayed P2.

(2) Inspiration ⇨ ↓intrathoracic pressure ⇨ ↑RV venous return ⇨ pulmonary pooling of blood ⇨ ↓ return to LV ⇨ ↓ LV ejection time ⇨ ↓ hangout interval ⇨ early A2.

- With expiration ⇨ the reverse occurs ⇨ early pulmonary valve closure ⇨ A2 - P2 interval separated by < 30 msec ⇨ single S2.

Expiratory splitting of S2 (Wide Split S2)

An expiratory split of S2 means that the A2 and P2 are separated by at least 30 - 40 msec.

Expiratory split means that the split is not only present during expiration, but it increases with inspiration.

Such an expiratory split is common in the recumbent position in young patients and children, but disappears or becomes single on sitting, standing or by Valsalva maneuver.

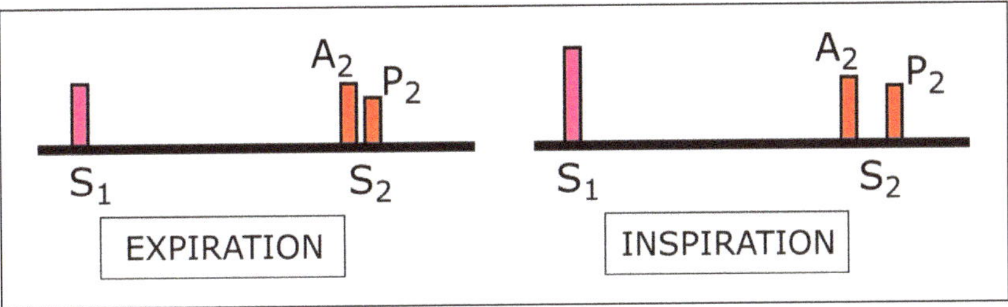

Fig. 10.2

However, presence of a persistent expiratory split, both in recumbent and sitting/standing positions is a very sensitive indicator of cardiac illnesses, RBBB being the most common cause.

Persistent expiratory splitting of the S2

Delayed P2 ⇨

- Delay in RV activation: RBBB, WPW syndrome, LV pacing, etc.
- Reduced impedance of the pulmonary vasculature (also ↑ hangout interval): ASD, PA dilatation, etc.
- Pressure overload of the RV (prolonged RV systole): RVF with PAH, PS, massive pulmonary embolism.

Early A2 ⇨

- ↓ LVOT resistance (short V systole): MR, constrictive pericarditis (also diastolic dysfunction), restrictive cardiomyopathy (also diastolic dysfunction).

> **NOTE**
>
> Expiratory splitting of S2 that is seen in cardiomyopathy occurs due to a combination of RV dysfunction, MR, ↓CO, bundle branch blocks, and PAH.

Wide split of S2 (described above)

By definition, it means the expiratory split of S2, and defined as wide if the split is audible in the standing posture in expiration.

Fixed splitting of S2

It means there is no change in the A2-P2 separation time during any phase of respiration.

ASD is a classical example of a wide and fixed split of S2.

Here the **split is wide** (described above) due to shunting of blood from the LA to the RA leading to ↑ RV filling that prolongs the RV systole, hence lengthening the hangout interval and delaying the P2 leading to the split.

The split is fixed because both the ventricles share a common venous reservoir due to which the inspiratory delay of the A2 and P2 equalizes.

Hence:

(1) During inspiration → ↑ venous return to the RA → no left to right shunt through ASD.

(2) During expiration → ↓ venous return to the RA → ↑ left to right shunting through the ASD → ↑ in both RV and LV filling→ no respiratory variation.

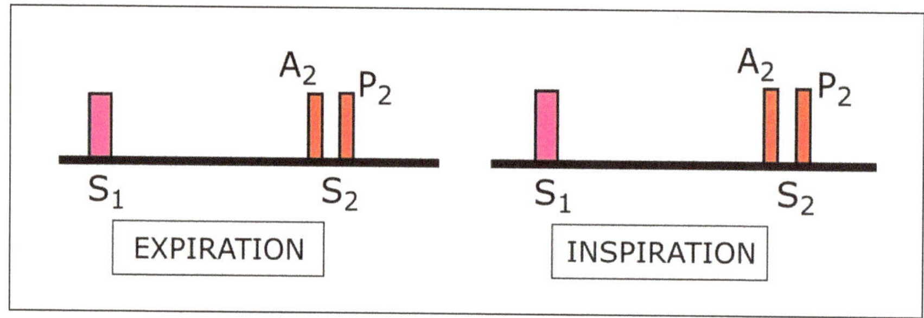

Fig. 10.3

A common approach to increase the A2 - P2 separation is to use the **Valsalva maneuver**.

In ASD, with Valsalva

→ Strain phase: continuous splitting

→ Release phase: A2 - P2 separation increases by < 0.02 seconds.

In normal subjects, splitting is ↑ in the release phase.

In ASD with Atrial fibrillation, the splitting ↑ during the longer cardiac cycles due to increased L → R shunting.

In normal subjects, there is no change in separation during the longer cycles.

Causes of wide fixed split of S2

→ ASD

→ Severe RV failure (RVF): RV doesn't respond to the ↑ volume during inspiration

→ TAPVC with ASD

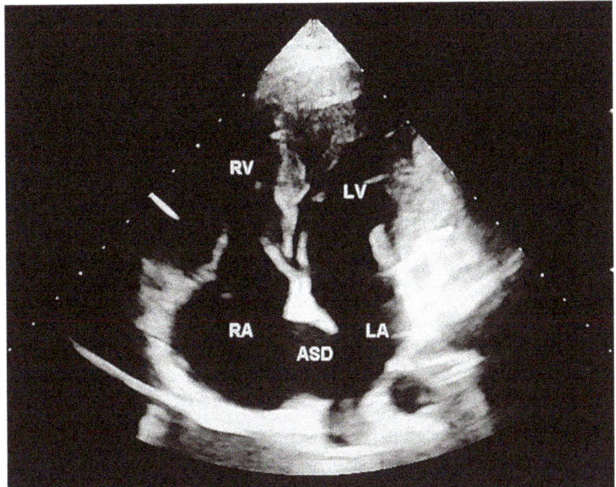

Fig. 10.4: Echocardiographic picture of an ASD.

Paradoxical/reversed splitting of S2

P2 occurs before A2 and the split is maximum in expiration and minimum/absent in inspiration (necessary criteria).

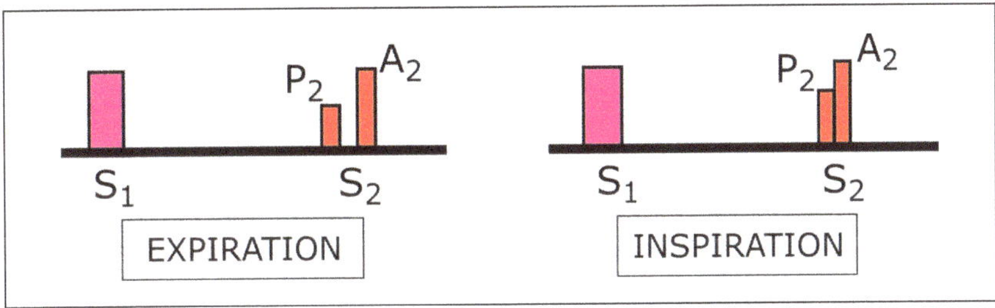

Fig. 10.5

Reversed splitting always indicates

→ CVS disease

→ Either delayed LV excitation or prolonged LV systole.

May occur due to delayed A2 or early P2.

Causes of delayed A2

→ Delayed LV excitation: Proximal LBBB (MC cause), pacing of the RV, RV ectopic beats.

→ Prolonged LV ejection: LVOT obstruction, severe AS, HOCM, acute MI, LV dysfunction, severe hypertension.

→ ↑ aortic hangout interval: Ascending aortic aneurysm, AS leading to post-stenotic dilatation, PDA.

Causes of early P2

→ WPW syndrome type B, right atrial myxoma, severe TR.

The spectrum of the paradoxical split of S2 depends on the extent of the delay in A2.

These could be:

→ A single S2

→ Complete paradoxical splitting

→ Incomplete paradoxical splitting (reversal confined only to expiration)

→ Paradoxical wide split

→ Paradoxical wide and fixed split

Clinically, the best method to identify the paradoxical split is to trace the A2 and P2 from the base (pulmonary area) to the apex. Normally, only the A2 can be traced from the base to the apex and P2 is heard only at the pulmonary area. But, when P2 is heard at the apex, a paradoxical split of the S2 is diagnosed clinically.

Pseudo Paradoxical split

In patients with thick chest wall or obese or having COPD, there could be a false disappearance of P2 on deep inspiration due to the expanding lungs interposing between the aorta and the stethoscope.

If the S2 happens to be split in expiration by any chance, then decreasing split or its disappearance in inspiration may wrongly give an impression of a paradoxical split of the S2 in such patients.

Distinguishing split S2 from other mimicking conditions

Clinically a split S2 may be confused with OS, S3, or pericardial knock.

(1) A2 - P2 split and A2 - OS

	A2 - P2 split	**A2 - OS**
Interval	Should be > 40 msec	30-150 msec
Site	Move from base to apex while auscultation	Mid precordium
Associated findings	Depends on the cause	S1 loud, and MDM of MS/TS
On standing	Remains same or sometimes narrows	Widens
With inspiration	Widens	Narrows

(2) A2 - P2 split and A2 - S3

	A2 - P2 split	A2 - S3
Interval	Should be > 40 msec	>150 msec
Site	Move from base to apex while auscultation	Apex
Frequency	High	Low
Associated findings	Depends on the cause	PSM of MR or TR

S3 occurs 0.14 - 0.16 seconds after the A2.

(3) Pericardial knock occurs 0.10 - 0.12 seconds after A2.

It is heard best at the apex.

It is similar to S3 but is slightly higher in pitch.

Single S2

Absent split in both the phases of respiration.

Common causes

⇨ Absence of A2: Severe AS, aortic atresia

⇨ Absence of P2: PS, TOF, pulmonary atresia, TGA (pulmonary artery is posterior)

⇨ Very loud P2: Severe PAH, Eisenmenger VSD (equal hangout intervals on both sides)

⇨ Presence of only one semilunar valve: Truncus arteriosus.

Intensity of the S2

Loud A2

⇨ Ascending aortic aneurysm (vascular dilatation)

⇨ Bicuspid aortic valve (mobile but thick leaflets)

⇨ Severe AR (↑valvular flow)

⇨ Hypertension (raised pressure distal to the valve)

⇨ Hyperdynamic states (↑valvular flow)

⇨ TGA (anteriorly placed aorta)

Soft A2

⇨ Sclerosed aortic valve

⇨ Calcified AS

Loud P2

⇨ Hyperdynamic states (↑valvular flow)

⇨ PAH

⇨ ASD (↑valvular flow)

⇨ Chest wall abnormalities (straight back syndrome) (due to close approximation of the heart to the chest wall)

⇨ Normal finding in infants and young children

Soft P2

⇨ Calcified PS

⇨ Obese patients due to thick chest wall, COPD

⇨ TGA, TOF, Pulmonary valve atresia, etc.

Clinically, the P2 is heard best at the pulmonary area but, the A2 is still louder than P2 at this area normally.

Loud P2 is said to be present if at the pulmonary area, P2 = A2 in intensity.

Loud P2 can be graded as:

⇨ Mild or (+1): P2 = A2

⇨ Moderate or (+2): P2 > A2

⇨ Severe or (+3): P2 >> A2 and banging in nature

A mildly loud P2 indicates a Pulmonary artery systolic pressure (PASP) of about 30-40 mmHg, moderately loud P2 indicates a PASP of about 40-70 mmHg, and a severely loud P2 indicates a PASP of > 70 mmHg.

References

- Synopsis of cardiac physical diagnosis; 2nd edition; Jonathan Abrams.
- Clinical examination in cardiology; 2nd edition; B N VIJAY RAGHAWA RAO.
- The art and science of cardiac physical examination; 2nd edition; Narasimhan Ranganathan.
- Clinical Methods: The History, Physical, and Laboratory Examinations. 3rd edition. Chapter 23 The Second Heart Sound by JOEL M. FELNER.
- Clinical methods in cardiology by B Soma Raju.
- Manual of practical medicine, 4th edition by R Alagappan.

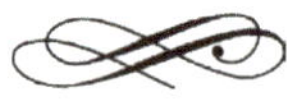

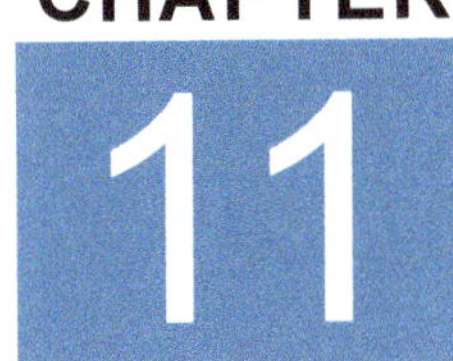

CHAPTER 11 The Third Heart Sound (S3)

The third heart sound is also called protodiastolic sound, ventricular diastolic gallop, S3 gallop, ventricular filling sound or early diastolic gallop.

It occurs in the early diastole at the end of the rapid filling phase of the ventricles.

Mechanism of S3 production

Any condition where there is a decrease in the early LV compliance can lead to a decrease in the LV/RV longitudinal lengthening during the rapid filling phase.

As such, when the mitral valve(or AV valves) opens, the blood column rushes from the LA to the LV but is decelerated suddenly due to the ↓ early LV compliance.

This deceleration produces vibrations within the entire CVS and also causes an impact of the heart with the anterior chest wall that leads to the production of S3.

Because S3 occurs at the end of the rapid filling phase

⇨ it coincides with the peak of the RF wave in apex cardiogram(described in the earlier chapters) and with the Y descent of the JVP for RVS3.

⇨ it is separated from S2 by the total time duration required for isovolumetric relaxation and the rapid filling phase (0.12 - 0.20 seconds after A2).

It is a low frequency sound (25 - 50 Hz) because it occurs at the end of the rapid filling phase where the majority of pressures are low.

With stenotic AV valves, S3 cannot be produced as the rapid filling of the ventricles cannot occur.

Normal characteristics of S3

Frequency: Low (25 - 50 HZ)

A2-S3 time interval: Physiological: 0.12 - 0.20 seconds

Pathological:- 0.14 - 0.16 seconds (occurs slightly early than physiological S3)

Auscultation: With the bell of the stethoscope with very light pressure

Best heard at

LVS3:- cardiac apex in left lateral decubitus with breath held in expiration. LVS3 intensity ↑ with isometric hand grip.

RVS3:- left lower sternum (or subxiphoid area) in supine position. RVS3 intensity ↑ on inspiration. It doesn't change with isometric hand grip.

Dynamic auscultation of S3

(1) Passive leg raising, sit ups, abdominal exercises, release phase of Valsalva → ↑venous return → ↑S3 intensity.

(2) Standing posture, strain phase of Valsalva → ↓venous return → ↓S3 intensity.

Physiological S3

(1) Common before the age of 40 years.

(2) Seen in children due to small heart size and rapid inflow that provides resistance.

(3) Pregnancy: since there is increased blood volume, circulation is rapid (high output state) and the sympathetic tone is increased.

(4) Anxiety

Pathological S3

The most important cause of pathological S3 is cardiac failure.

S3 means "a failing heart"

S4 means "a straining heart"

Causes of pathological S3

⇨ LV/RV failure: high filling pressures

⇨ Ventricular dysfunction: IHD, cardiomyopathies, myocarditis, cor pulmonale, hypertension.

⇨ Hyperdynamic circulation: beri beri, hyperthyroidism, IV fluid, anaemia, renal failure, AV fistula.

⇨ Regurgitant lesions (MR, TR, AR, TR): large v waves with rapid pressure reversal during ventricular dilatation.

⇨ Congenital heart diseases:

- ASD, VSD, PDA - due to ventricular overload.
- TAPVC, truncus arteriosus, TGA with VSD - due to ↑ pulmonary blood flow.

⇨ Constrictive pericarditis: ↑ pressure in the atria and venous system.

NOTE

Ebstein's anomaly, severe PS with normal ventricular septum, R→L atrial shunt with heart failure are some congenital heart diseases with ↓ pulmonary blood flow, but shows S3.

If S3 is absent in a case of heart failure then one must suspect

- ⇨ Cardiac tamponade
- ⇨ MS
- ⇨ TS
- ⇨ MI with LVF

The presence or absence of S3 divides shock into cardiogenic or non-cardiogenic.

Etiologies of shock with no S3 are

- ⇨ Shock due to hypovolemia
- ⇨ Shock due to septicemia
- ⇨ Pericardial effusion with tamponade
- ⇨ Tension pneumothorax

Clinical auscultation of S3

The left lateral decubitus position is important for auscultation of S3. Patient should hold the breath in expiration for proper hearing of S3. It is a very low frequency sound hence, the room should be very silent without even the slightest of noise.

Ideally, for auscultation of S3, we start from the pulmonary area where we pay attention to S2 and the time interval after that. Usually, the post-S2 time interval(diastole) is very quiet in the pulmonary area. Having done with this post-S2 time interval at the pulmonary area, we keep moving our stethoscope slowly towards the apex paying full attention to any new sound that occurs after S2. By this method, there is a high chance that we successfully detect any S3 occuring there.

NOTE

- ⇨ LVS3 may be physiological/pathological
- ⇨ RVS3- always pathological
- ⇨ LVS3 indicates a LVEDP > 25 mmHg.

Table 11.2: Differences between A2 - OS and A2 - S3

	A2 - OS	A2 - S3
Site	Mid Precordium (between left sternal border and apex)	Apex
Time	0.03-0.15 seconds	0.12-0.20 seconds
Pitch	Medium to high	Very low
Contour	Snapping	Thudding
Associated with	S1 loud, MDM of MS/TS	Features of LVF, PSM of MR/TR
On standing	Increases	Remains the same

Differences between S3 and tumour plop

Many times, tumor plop may mimic S3.

However, tumor plop has a loud and banging M1 as an association.

It is also associated with a mitral obstructive diastolic murmur which may be of low to medium frequency.

Tumor plop occurs 0.08 - 0.13 seconds after the S2.

References

- Synopsis of cardiac physical diagnosis; 2nd edition; Jonathan Abrams.
- Clinical examination in cardiology; 2nd edition; B N VIJAY RAGHAWA RAO.
- The art and science of cardiac physical examination; 2nd edition; Narasimhan Ranganathan.
- Clinical Methods: The History, Physical, and Laboratory Examinations. 3rd edition. Chapter 24 The Third Heart Sound by MARK E. SILVERMAN.
- Clinical methods in cardiology by B Soma Raju.
- Manual of practical medicine, 4th edition by R Alagappan.

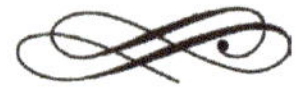

CHAPTER

12 The Fourth Heart Sound (S4)

The fourth heart sound or S4 is also known as “atrial gallop”, “presystolic gallop” or “late diastolic sound”.

Although called as atrial gallop, it is actually a ventricular sound.

The primary requirements for the production of S4 includes:

- ↓compliance of the ventricles (stiff ventricle)
- Normal functioning atrium
- Normal sinus rhythm
- Normal AV valves

Mechanism of production of S4

In a normal heart, atrial contraction in the terminal phase of diastole contributes to 15% of the ventricular filling.

However, when the ventricle is noncompliant, the atrial contraction contributes upto 25% of the ventricular filling and tries to pump the blood in the ventricles with great force. But because the ventricle is stiff with a raised end diastolic pressure, there is a sudden deceleration of the incoming blood in the late phase of diastole that sets vibrations in the ventricular wall along with a dynamic thrust of the heart to the anterior chest wall. All these things collectively lead to the production of S4. An important point to note here is that a strong atrial contraction is necessary for the production of S4.

Normal characteristics of S4

Frequency: Low (20 - 30 Hz)

Auscultation: With the bell of the stethoscope with light pressure

Best heard at

- LVS4: at the apex in left lateral decubitus position in expiration
- RVS4: at the lower left sternum in supine position in inspiration

Dynamic auscultation

⇨ Sustained handgrip, exercise → ↑venous return → increased intensity of LVS4 and increased separation from S2.

⇨ Upright position → ↓venous return and sympathetic tachycardia → decreased intensity of LVS4 and decreased separation from S2, sometimes merging with the S2.

Hemodynamic correlations

⇨ LVS4 indicates a LVEDP > 15 mmHg, follows the P wave in ECG by 0.14-0.20 seconds, and precedes the S1.

⇨ RVS4 indicates a RVEDP > 12 mmHg, and coincides with a prominent a wave in JVP.

Causes of S4

Physiological

⇨ > 60 years of age: due to age related ventricular hypertrophy and sometimes asymptomatic IHDs.

Pathological

⇨ ***Increased late diastolic phase***

- Hyperdynamic circulation: Hyperthyroidism, AV fistula, etc.
- Acute regurgitant lesions like MR, AR, TR: where the LA is loaded with blood and the ventricles do not get appropriate time to dilate due to acuteness of the disease

⇨ ***Impaired ventricular compliance***

- Severe AS (indicates a peak systolic gradient > 74 mmHg), HOCM, Hypertension, etc.
- Severe Pulmonary stenosis (RVEDP > 12 mmHg)
- Acute coronary syndrome: MI (indicates that at least 10% of the myocardium is damaged and LVEDP > 18mmHg), angina pectoris, etc.
- Heart blocks: 1^0,2^0,3^0.

S4 doesn't occur with

(1) Chronic MR ⇨ as the ventricles dilate over a long time and become compliant.

(2) Non sinus rhythm (Atrial fibrillation) ⇨ due to no proper atrial contraction.

(3) Stenotic AV lesions ⇨ there is obstruction to atrial contraction force

(4) Unhealthy atrium ⇨ no proper atrial contraction force

References

- Synopsis of cardiac physical diagnosis; 2nd edition; Jonathan Abrams.
- Clinical examination in cardiology; 2nd edition; B N VIJAY RAGHAWA RAO.
- The art and science of cardiac physical examination; 2nd edition; Narasimhan Ranganathan.
- Clinical Methods: The History, Physical, and Laboratory Examinations. 3rd edition.Chapter 25 The Fourth Heart Sound by ERIC S. WILLIAMS.
- Clinical methods in cardiology by B Soma Raju.

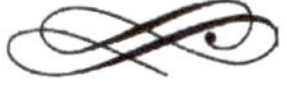

CHAPTER

13 Other Heart Sounds

PERICARDIAL KNOCK (PK)

→ Seen characteristically in chronic constrictive pericarditis where the heart is surrounded by a thick, fibrous pericardium, sometimes calcified.

→ PK is similar to S3 but occurs slightly earlier and has a slightly higher intensity.

→ It is an early diastolic sound and occurs due to sudden stoppage of the diastolic ventricular filling due to thick pericardium.

→ It occurs around 0.09 - 0.12 seconds after A2.

→ Best heard along the left lower sternal border and ↑ on deep inspiration.

→ Usually associated with other features like ↑JVP, Friedreich's sign, Kussmaul's sign, Square root sign, etc that helps to distinguish it from the OS of MS.

Square Root Sign ⇨

In chronic constrictive pericarditis, the pressure inside the ventricles during diastole rises suddenly to very high levels and then plateau or remains the same until end diastole which produces the classical SQUARE-ROOT SIGN on recording the ventricular pressure curves.

TUMOR PLOP

→ Tumor plop is a high frequency sound characteristically seen in atrial myxomas.

→ Atrial myxoma is common in LA but can also occur in RA. They are usually pedunculated with a long stalk attached to the atrial septum.

→ These myxomas usually sit on the AV valve orifice during diastole and produce either mitral valve or tricuspid valve obstructive features, which corresponds to a prominent v wave in LA pressure tracings (due to ↑LAP) and prominent a wave and rapid y descent in RA pressure tracings (JVP).

→ Once the AV valves open during the rapid filling phase, this Tumor protrudes into the ventricle rapidly and is abruptly stopped once the maximum excursion is reached which produces the Tumor plop.

→ It usually occurs 0.08 - 0.13 seconds after the S2.

→ May be associated with a mitral obstructive diastolic murmur which may be of low to medium frequency.

→ A loud and banging M1 may be present due to the raised LAP.

→ The symptoms of the patient may be related to the body position because gravity may cause the Tumor to sit on the AV valve once the patient assumes an erect posture.→ NAME syndrome: nevi, atrial myxoma, myxoid neurofibroma, ephelides.

→ LAMB syndrome: lentigines, atrial myxoma, blue nevi.

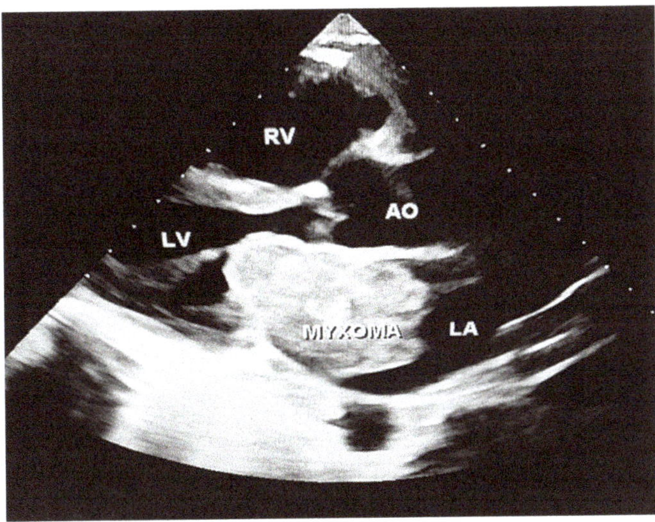

Fig. 13.1: A large LA myxoma.

OPENING SNAP (OS)

Opening snap (OS) is a high frequency, early diastolic, clicking sound caused by the sudden stoppage of the opening AV valves, especially when the valve leaflets are thick and deformed but mobile and is associated with an ↑ LAP or ↑ flow across the valves.

For all of our practical purposes, we use the word OS in context to mitral stenosis where OS occurs due to doming movement of the thickened mitral leaflets towards the LV because of an ↑ LAP.

Characteristics of Opening snap

Frequency: High

Occurs in: Early diastole following A2 after an average interval of about 60-120 ms.

Auscultation: With the diaphragm of the stethoscope just inside of the apex beat for Mitral OS and lower left sternum for Tricuspid OS. The mitral OS is better heard after exercise and it does not change with respiration. The OS is usually followed by the MDM which becomes prominent with exercise.

NOTE

The mitral OS may sometimes be heard at the pulmonary area and may be confused with a split S2.

Etiopathogenesis of OS

(1) **AV valve stenosis** ⇨ MS, TS

(2) **↑Flow across the AV valves with great force** ⇨

Mitral valve: MR, large VSD, HOCM, MVP, hyperthyroidism, PDA.

Tricuspid valve: Large ASD, TR, Ebstein anomaly.

Conditions where OS can be missed even in the presence of a significant MS

⇨ Very severely calcified, immobile mitral valves

⇨ Severe MR

⇨ Severe AR

⇨ Severe AS

⇨ LV dysfunction or LVF with CAD

⇨ When OS is heard at the pulmonary area, where it is misinterpreted as a split S2.

The A2 - OS interval

Now, thinking of the sequences of the cardiac cycle, we know:-

With the end of systole → beginning of isovolumetric relaxation (diastole) → closure of the aortic valve(A2) → LA - LV pressure crossover (where LA pressure exceeds LV pressure) → opening of the mitral valve (to produce OS).

From the above sequence, it is clear that it is the LAP that can influence the MV opening time. If the LAP is raised, the LA - LV pressure crossover time is reduced and the MV opens immediately following the A2, i.e.; the A2 - OS time decreases.

Since the LAP increases with the increasing severity of MS, the A2 - OS interval has an inverse relation to the MS severity.........more the severity of MS, lesser is the A2 - OS interval and vice versa.

Although the A2 - OS interval also depends on the aortic pressure level, and the rate of isovolumetric relaxation, the LAP is the most important factor that influences the A2 - OS interval.

The normal A2 - OS interval ranges between 50-120 ms.

In mild MS: A2 - OS interval is > 120 ms with a rough LAP of around 14-15 mmHg.

In moderate MS: A2 - OS interval is around 80 - 100 ms with a rough LAP of around 20 - 22 mmHg.

In severe MS: A2 - OS interval is around 50 - 70 ms with a rough LAP of around 24 - 25 mmHg.

However, there are numerous factors that can affect the A2 - OS interval. Some of them are enumerated below:-

(1) Heart rate (HR):

↑HR ⇨ ↓A2 - OS interval because of the shortened diastole.

↓HR ⇨ ↑A2 - OS interval because of the prolonged diastole.

(2) Time of aortic closure (occurrence of A2):

Hypertension ⇨ ↑A2 - OS interval because of early A2.

AS ⇨ ↓A2 - OS interval because of delayed A2.

AR ⇨ ↑A2 - OS interval because of early A2.

(3) Low LAP:

↑A2 - OS interval as seen in RV dysfunction, TR, PAH, etc.

(4) ↑LA - LV pressure crossover time (↑LVEDP):

↑A2 - OS interval in conditions like IHD, LV dysfunction in cardiomyopathies, etc.

Table 13.1: Differences between A2 - OS and A2 - P2

	A2 - OS	**A2 - P2**
Best heard at	Just inside the apex	Pulmonary area
Time interval	50 - 120 ms	< 30 ms
Posture effect	Widens on standing	Narrows on standing
Respiratory variation	No change for mitral OS	Widens on inspiration

EJECTION CLICKS (EC)

Ejection clicks (EC) also known as systolic ejection sounds (SES) are high pitched sounds occurring in early systole and follow S1.

EC is a true indicator of an underlying CVS disease and reflects that a particular systolic murmur (SM) is actually organic in nature.

They can originate from either side of the heart.

NOTE

Opening snap (OS) is the diastolic counterpart of ejection systolic clicks.

Ejection sounds can originate from:

⇨ Aortic or pulmonary valves where they are called valvular ejection clicks. Usually associated with a soft S2.

⇨ Dilated great arterial roots where they are called non-valvular or vascular ejection clicks or sounds. Usually associated with a loud S2.

Theories of production of EC:

⇨ Valvular ejection clicks occur due to doming and sudden halt of motion of the thickened, stenotic, but mobile leaflets during early systole (EC do not occur with valve calcification).

⇨ Vascular ejection clicks occur due to sudden stretching and reverberations of the proximally dilated great arteries which usually have a raised systolic pressure and poor compliance.

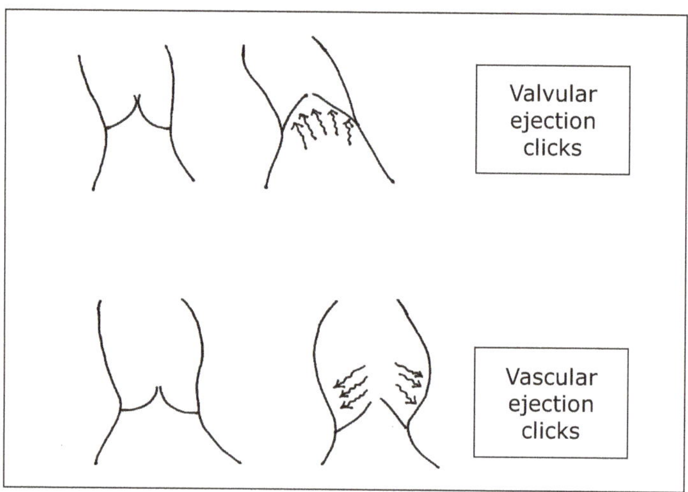

Fig. 13.2

Valvular ejection clicks

Aortic

⇨ Usually follows the S1 by 40 - 50 msec.

⇨ High frequency sound

⇨ Coincides with the initial carotid upstroke

⇨ Best heard with the diaphragm of the stethoscope at the right 2nd ICS or the apex with the patient comfortably seated and leaned forward.

⇨ Aortic valvular click heard only at the apex: eldery, and chronic pulmonary diseases.

⇨ Does not vary with respiration as the LVEDP is always < than the aortic pressure in diastole.

- ⇨ Characteristically seen in congenital aortic valve stenosis.
- ⇨ More severe the stenosis, earlier is the click.
- ⇨ Not seen with sub valvular or supra valvular stenosis of the aorta.
- ⇨ May be associated with pulsus parvus, LVH, soft or absent A2, systolic thrill at the neck, etc.

Pulmonary

- ⇨ High frequency sound
- ⇨ Coincides with the pulmonary pressure curve upstroke.
- ⇨ Best heard with the diaphragm of the stethoscope at the left 2nd ICS or the left sternal border with the patient seated comfortably and leaned forward.
- ⇨ Better heard in expiration and diminishes or disappears in inspiration.
- ⇨ With PS→RVH and RV stiffening→with inspiration→↑venous return→↑RVEDP→partial and premature opening of the pulmonary valve(PV) in diastole→when RV contracts→the already partially opened PV produces a softer and early occurring click.
- ⇨ With severe valvular type PS, the RV becomes so much stiff that even atrial contraction leads to complete opening of the PV leading to a late diastolic click. More the severity of PS, the closer it is to the S1.
- ⇨ This is the only right sided cardiac event that ↓ on inspiration.
- ⇨ May be associated with prominent a waves, widely split S2, etc.

Vascular/Nonvalvular ejection clicks

Aortic

- ⇨ High frequency
- ⇨ Does not radiate from the aortic area
- ⇨ May be associated with a loud S2

Pulmonary

- ⇨ High frequency
- ⇨ Heard at the left 2nd ICS in inspiration.
- ⇨ The click may be palpable over the PA.
- ⇨ Loud P2
- ⇨ Narrow split S2

Etiology

Aortic valvular click

- ⇨ Congenital aortic valvular stenosis
- ⇨ Bicuspid and quadricuspid aortic valves

Pulmonary valvular click

- ⇨ Pulmonary valve stenosis
- ⇨ TOF

Aortic vascular click

- ⇨ Hypertension
- ⇨ AR
- ⇨ Ascn aortic aneurysm
- ⇨ Hyperdynamic states like anemia, hyperthyroidism, etc.
- ⇨ TOF

Pulmonary vascular click

- ⇨ Pulmonary artery dilatation
- ⇨ PAH
- ⇨ ASD
- ⇨ Hyperdynamic states

NOTE

- ⇨ Beyond 40 years of age, AS is bound to get calcified. Hence, aortic valvular click in such a patient indicates a milder form of AS.
- ⇨ Aortic valvular click better heard at the apex can be easily confused with a possible loud S1. However, a loud S1 better heard at the base than at the apex would indicate a click and a loud S1.

- ⇨ **EC can be confused sometimes with S4 - S1.**

  Points favouring S4 - S1 are

  - S4 - S1 heard with the bell of the stethoscope with light pressure
  - LVS4 heard at apex, RVS4 heard at the left lower sternal border
  - Features of LVH may be there.
  - Inspiration will ↑ the intensity of RVS4.

⇨ **Distinguishing features of split S1 from EC**

- Split S1 does not radiate to any other area apart from the apex.
- The T1 component is not heard at the base.

NON EJECTION SOUNDS/SYSTOLIC CLICKS (SC)

Systolic clicks are high frequency sounds that occur at the AV valve levels and are mostly related to prolapse of the mitral (more common) or tricuspid valves, most commonly caused due to myxomatous degeneration.

In mitral valve prolapse (MVP) syndrome, the valve leaflets prolapse inside the LA during systole which produces the click.

Normally the chordae and papillary muscles give support to the MV leaflets and prevent their prolapse.

In disease states like myxomatous degeneration, the chordae becomes long and superfluous and the papillary muscle malfunctions which causes the leaflets to prolapse into the LA with sudden tensing of the chordae during systole producing the click.

Similarly, there can be multiple clicks if different chordae are tensed at slightly different times.

Many times, the SC of MVP is associated with the systolic murmur of MR also.

The degree (intensity of SC) and time of leaflet prolapse, i.e.; the S1-SC interval is determined by the LV volume at end diastole and the force of ejection.

Any maneuver that ↓ LV volume at end diastole will make the click louder and earlier (closer to S1 or S1-SC interval ↓) and vice versa. This is because when the LV volume increases, the LV size is also increased that causes the chordae to stretch and hence the prolapse decreases.

Characteristics of mitral valve Systolic click

Frequency: High

Timing with systole: Mid- to late systolic, occurs approximately 0.14 seconds after S1.

Auscultation: Heard with the diaphragm of the stethoscope.

Best heard at: Apex for MVP click.

Left lower sternal border for TVP click.

Dynamic auscultation and maneuvers

(1) Standing, Phase II Valsalva, NTG, Inhalation of amyl nitrate → ↓LV size and volume at end diastole → early (↓S1-SC interval) and loud intensity SC.

(2) Prompt squatting, hand grip, Phase IV Valsalva, supine posture, vasopressors like phenyl epinephrine → ↑LV size and volume at end diastole → delayed (↑S1-SC interval) and low intensity or absent SC.

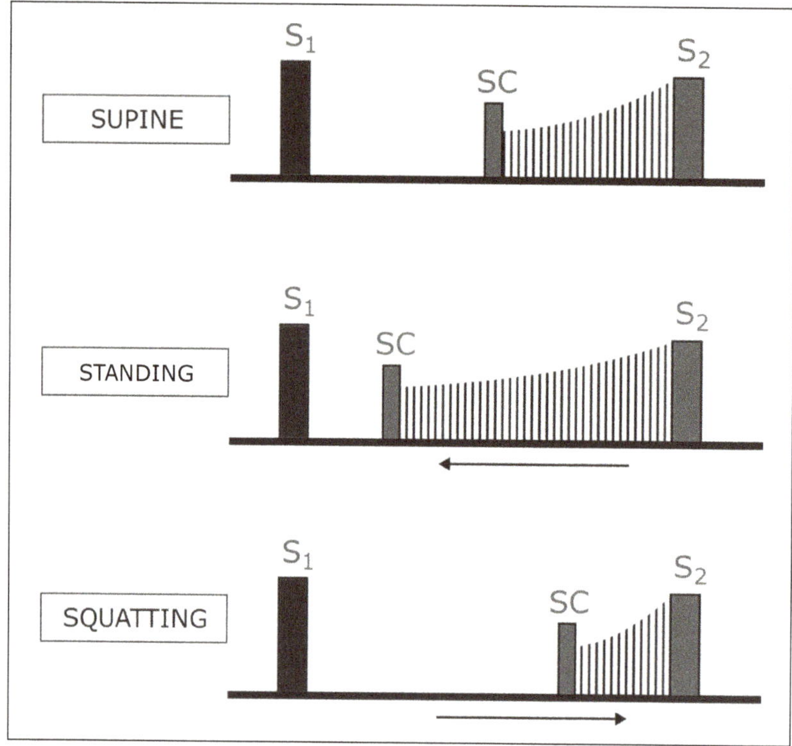

Fig. 13.3: MVP systolic click (SC) changes with changes of body posture.

PROSTHETIC VALVE SOUNDS

Prosthetic valve sounds are important to know because they have their own auscultatory findings due to all the motions involved and changes in the flow pattern.

Different types of prosthetic devices can produce different intensity sounds which can be influenced by the cardiac rhythm and hemodynamic changes.

Prosthetic valves can have their own closing and opening sounds and can be associated with systolic or diastolic murmurs.

Prosthetic valve sounds are heard with the help of diaphragm of the stethoscope since they are high frequency sounds or clicks.

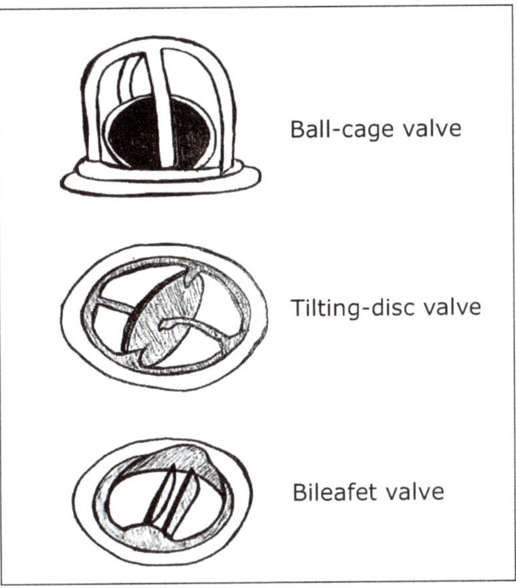

Fig. 13.4

(1) Ball valve/Ball-in-cage prosthesis (Starr-Edwards, Smeloff- Cutter, McGovern)

⇨ **Mitral**

- Most widely known and studied prosthetic valve.
- Mitral opening sound (MOS) follows the A2 by about 0.07 - 0.11 seconds.
- MOS best heard at the apex.
- MOS intensity is normally > mitral closure sound (MCS) which is best heard at the left lower sternal border.
- A2 - MOS interval < 0.05 seconds suggests prosthetic obstruction or severe MR and interval > 0.17 seconds suggests abnormalities of the poppet movement.
- Low intensity MCS → 1^0 heart blocks.
- Absent MOS → after a premature beat.
- Early- or mid- SM at left lower sternal border → normal finding due to turbulence.
- Diastolic murmur → suggests obstruction.

⇨ **Aortic**

- Aortic opening click (sound) (AOS) intensity is > aortic closure sound (ACS).
- A1-AOS interval is about 0.07 second.
- AOS → apex or left lower sternal border.
- ↓ cardiac output → ↓ intensity of sounds
- ↑ HR and anemia → ↑ intensity of sounds.

- Absent AOS → prosthetic dysfunction.
- Systolic ejection murmur upto grade 2 or 3 out of 6 is a normal finding.
- Diastolic murmur → abnormal finding.

(2) Disk valves (Bjork-Shiley)

⇨ **Mitral**

- Only MCS is heard.
- No opening sound is heard because these are very lightweight disks that do not hit any resonant structure(s), although opening sounds can be recorded only by phonocardiograms. The A2-opening sound interval is about 0.05 - 0.09 seconds.
- MCS is best heard at the apex.
- Absent or soft MCS → LV dysfunction, 1^{0} heart block, thrombosis, fibrosis.
- MSM → normal finding upto grade 2/6.
- Diastolic murmur due to turbulence is a normal finding.

⇨ **Aortic**

- AOS is not heard with the stethoscope but can be recorded by a phonocardiogram. The M1-AOS interval is about 0.04 seconds.
- Absent ACS → thrombus, LV dysfunction.
- Mid systolic ejection murmur → normal finding.

(3) Tissue valves (Porcine valves)

⇨ **Mitral**

- MOS is best heard at apex, and occurs 0.07 - 0.11 seconds after A2.
- MCS is best heard at the left lower sternal border.
- Diastolic murmur is abnormal and indicates suture disruption, infection, and thrombosis.

⇨ **Aortic**

- Only ACS is heard, best at aortic and pulmonary areas.
- 2/6 MSM is a normal finding along the left lower sternal border.
- Diastolic murmur is an abnormal finding.

(4) Bivalve prosthesis (St. Jude's)

⇨ **Mitral**

- Both MOS, and MCS heard.

⇨ **Aortic**

- AOS heard due to turbulent flow.

- ACS coincides with the carotid pulse dicrotic notch.
- Occasional early SM is a normal finding.
- Diastolic murmur is an abnormal finding.

PERICARDIAL FRICTION RUB (PR)

Pericardial friction rub is a high frequency, superficial and scratchy sound which can be heard over the precordium in patients of acute pericarditis.

It is thought to be produced due to rubbing or friction between the two layers of the inflamed pericardium, but it does not explain the pericardial rub occurring in patients of large pericardial effusions.

The prevalence of PR in acute pericarditis ranges between 35 - 85% and 15.2% in chronic pericardial diseases.

The PR is nearly 100% specific for an acute pericarditis.

The classic PR is high pitched and has a scratchy, leather quality.

Auscultated with the diaphragm of the stethoscope best at the left lower sternal border with the patient seated and leaned forward or in the knee-elbow position with the breath held in expiration.

It can change with posture.

Sometimes, a pleural rub may be interpreted as a PR. In such cases, we ask the patient to hold his breath. If it is a pleural rub, it will disappear.

A classical pericardial rub is TRIPHASIC which indicates the movement of the heart inside the pericardium in atrial systole, ventricular systole and the rapid filling phases.

Thus, atrial fibrillation will produce only 1 or 2 phases of the PR.

European Society of Cardiology (2015) criteria for acute pericarditis(at least 2 criteria required)

⇨ pericardial chest pain

⇨ pericardial rub

⇨ ECG changes - diffuse ST-elevation or PR-depression

⇨ pericardial effusion (new onset or worsening).

Causes of acute pericarditis

⇨ Infective, especially tuberculosis

⇨ Uremia

⇨ MI (acute)

⇨ Cardiothoracic surgery

⇨ Rheumatic fever

⇨ Mediastinal irradiation

NOTE

Means-Lerman scratch is a type of sound which is commonly confused with pericardial rub.

It is commonly heard in hyperthyroidism which is a hyperdynamic state leading to friction of the pericardium with the pleura leading to a scratchy mid-systolic sound.

It is best heard at the pulmonary area or the upper part of the sternum in forced expiration.

MEDIASTINAL CRUNCH

Mediastinal crunch are high frequency, scratchy sounds or clicks during ventricular contraction phase seen in pneumomediastinum.

These sounds are heard commonly over the cardiac apex or left lower sternal border.

They occur in synchrony with the heart beats.

Also called **"Hamman's sign"** in pneumomediastinum.

70% of patients with pneumomediastinum have Subcutaneous emphysema.

References

- Burgess TE, Le NN, Olds GS, et al. BMJ Case Rep 2019;12:e233546. doi:10.1136/bcr-2019- 233546 Pericardial knock.
- Synopsis of cardiac physical diagnosis; 2nd edition; Jonathan Abrams.
- Clinical examination in cardiology; 2nd edition; B N VIJAY RAGHAWA RAO.
- The art and science of cardiac physical examination; 2nd edition; Narasimhan Ranganathan.
- Clinical Methods: The History, Physical, and Laboratory Examinations. 3rd edition.Chapter 25 The Fourth Heart Sound by ERIC S. WILLIAMS.
- Clinical methods in cardiology by B Soma Raju.
- Clinical examination in cardiology; 2nd edition; B N VIJAY RAGHAWA RAO.
- The art and science of cardiac physical examination; 2nd edition; Narasimhan Ranganathan.

- Br Heart J: first published as 10.1136/hrt.15.2.135 on 1 April 1953. THE OPENING SNAP OF MITRAL STENOSIS BY PATRICK MOUNSEY.
- Clinical examination in cardiology; 2nd edition; B N VIJAY RAGHAWA RAO.
- The art and science of cardiac physical examination; 2nd edition; Narasimhan Ranganathan.
- Clinical methods in cardiology by B Soma Raju.
- Synopsis of cardiac physical diagnosis; 2nd edition; Jonathan Abrams.
- Clinical examination in cardiology; 2nd edition; B N VIJAY RAGHAWA RAO.
- Clinical Methods: The History, Physical, and Laboratory Examinations. 3rd edition Chapter28 Ejection Clicks by WILLIAM R. JACOBS.
- Clinical methods in cardiology by B Soma Raju.
- Clinical examination in cardiology; 2nd edition; B N VIJAY RAGHAWA RAO.
- Clinical methods in cardiology by B Soma Raju.
- Annals of Internal Medicine. 1981;95:594-598. Auscultation of the Normally Functioning Prosthetic Valve by NEALE D. SMITH, M.D.; VEENA RAIZADA, M.D.; and JONATHAN ABRAMS, M.D.
- Clinical examination in cardiology; 2nd edition; B N VIJAY RAGHAWA RAO.
- Chahine J, Siddiqui WJ. Pericardial Friction Rub. [Updated 2019 May 13]. In: StatPearls [Internet]. Treasure Island (FL): StatPearls Publishing; 2020 Pericardial Friction Rub.
- Circulation. 2006;113:1622-1632. Pericardial Disease by William C. Little, MD; Gregory L. Freeman, MD.
- Am Fam Physician 2007;76:1509-14 Acute Pericarditis by LESLIE E. TINGLE, MD; DANIEL MOLINA, MD; and CHARLES W. CALVERT, DO.
- J Thorac Dis. 2015 Feb; 7(Suppl 1): S44–S49. Pneumomediastinum by Vasileios K. Kouritas, Konstantinos Papagiannopoulos, George Lazaridis, Sofia Baka, Ioannis Mpoukovinas, Vasilis Karavasilis, Sofia Lampaki, Ioannis Kioumis, Georgia Pitsiou, Antonis Papaiwannou, Anastasia Karavergou, Maria Kipourou, Martha Lada, John Organtzis, Nikolaos Katsikogiannis, Kosmas Tsakiridis, Konstantinos Zarogoulidis, and Paul Zarogoulidis.

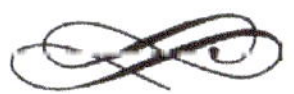

CHAPTER

14 Cardiac Murmurs

Cardiac murmurs are audible vibrations produced due to turbulence of the blood flow which in turn is determined by the blood flow velocity and the area of the opening through which it flows (where the Reynolds number goes > 2000).

The mechanisms responsible for cardiac murmur production are

- ⇨ ↑rate of flow of blood through normal or diseased orifice.
- ⇨ flow of blood from a narrow opening into a dilated chamber/vessel.
- ⇨ regurgitation through a diseased valve.
- ⇨ shunting of blood

Clinical evaluation of a cardiac murmur

It is very obvious that for a proper recognition of a cardiac murmur, we need to have its detailed evaluation and study it with respect to:

- ⇨ Timing (systolic/diastolic/continuous)
- ⇨ Place or location of best audibility/intensity
- ⇨ Length/duration
- ⇨ Grade/loudness
- ⇨ Pitch
- ⇨ Shape/configuration
- ⇨ Radiation to other site
- ⇨ Dynamic auscultation

TIME OF THE MURMUR

Here we try to detect whether the murmur is a systolic, diastolic or a continuous murmur.

(1) Systolic

Murmur starts at or just after S1, but ending before S2 (this can be checked by palpating the carotid upstroke and apex thrust that occurs immediately after S1, discussed in earlier chapters).

Systolic murmurs are further sub-classified as:-

- ⇨ **Early systolic (ESM):** Starts with S1 and ending before mid-systole. Usually decrescendo in configuration.

⇨ **Mid systolic (MSM):** Starts after S1 and and ending before respective A2 or P2, i.e.; S2. Also called ejection systolic murmur. Has crescendo-decrescendo type of configuration (diamond shaped murmurs).

↑ejection→murmur↑.

↓ejection→murmur↓.

⇨ **Late systolic (LSM):** Usually begins after ejection and terminates at or before S2. High pitched murmurs.

⇨ **Pan- or Holosystolic (PSM):** Occupies the whole period from S1 to S2 due to a wide difference in pressures between two cardiac chambers like LV→LA or LV→RV.

Examples are VSD, MR, TR.

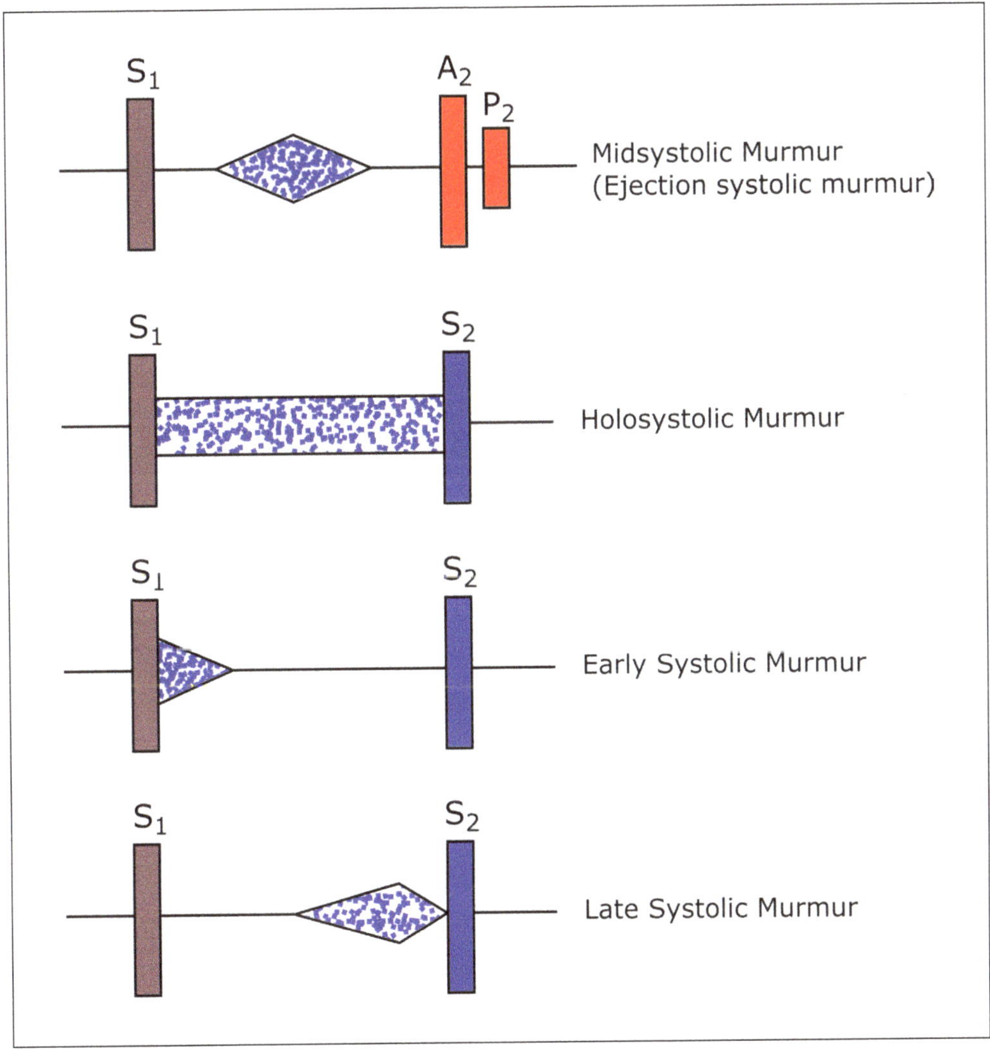

Fig. 14.1

(2) Diastolic

Murmur starts at or just after S2, but ending before the next S1.

Diastolic murmurs are further sub-classified as:-

⇨ **Early diastolic (EDM):** Starts at or just after S2. Usually associated with fall of ventricular pressures below the great arteries (aorta or PA). Usually high pitched, with a blowing and decrescendo character.

⇨ **Mid diastolic (MDM):** Starts after S2 and stops before S1. Usually low pitched and associated with diseased AV valves(mitral and tricuspid) when there is a discrepency between AV valve area and the ventricular diastolic blood flow. However, sometimes even normal AV valves can have MDM when the diastolic blood flow is increased, e.g.; VSD, PDA, ASD.

⇨ **Late diastolic (LDM)/Presystolic:** Occurs just before S1 during the rapid ventricular filling phase preceded by the atrial contraction. Usually associated with MS or TS but, sometimes also seen with atrial myxomas.

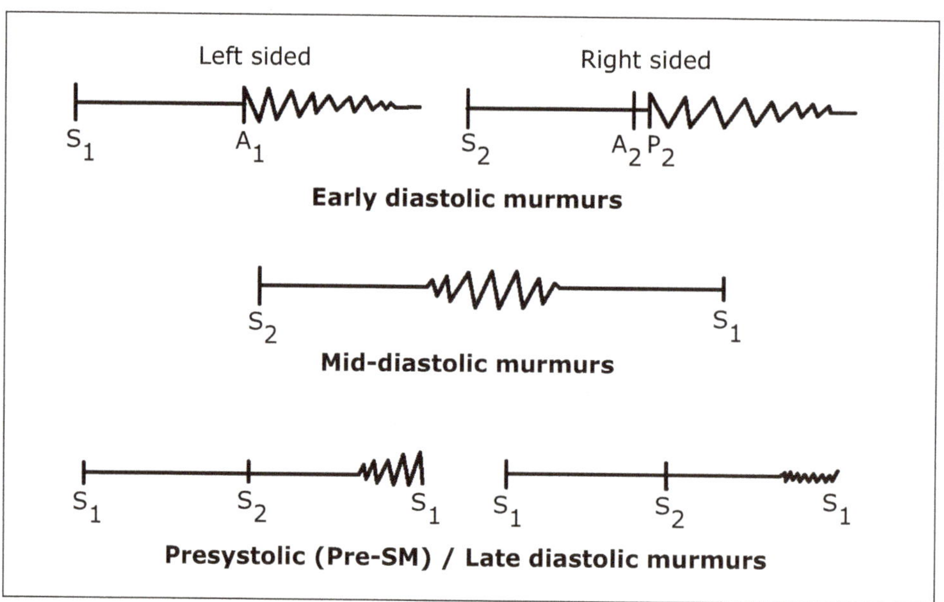

Fig. 14.2

(3) Continuous murmur (CM): A murmur that occupies the whole of systole and diastole with a constant character. Care must be taken not to misinterpret a combination of systolic and diastolic murmur(mixed stenotic and regurgitant lesion) as a CM.

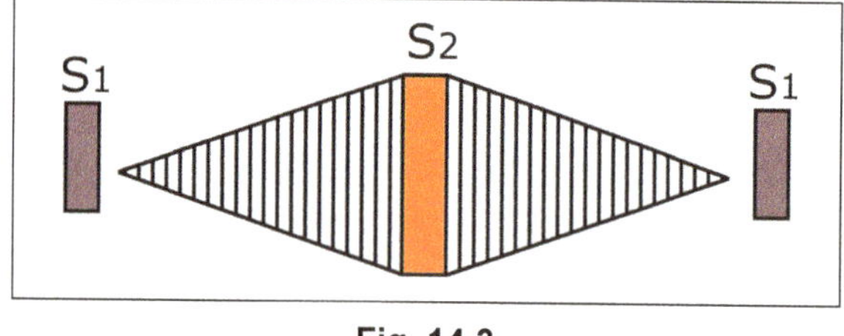

Fig. 14.3

Location of the murmur

Location or site of the murmur means the place where it is best heard. Usually, a murmur is heard in >1 area. But we should have an idea about the place where it can be best heard.

Example: the MDM of MS can sometimes be also heard at the tricuspid area (TA) and the lower left sternal border (LLSB).

Murmurs heard at cardiac apex area

⇨ **Only cardiac apex:** Mid diastolic murmur in MS, ↑Diastolic flow murmur in MR, ESM in AS with valve calcification with emphysema (since only the LV apex is exposed) (also called Gallavardin effect).

⇨ **Can be heard at cardiac apex:** EDM in aortic regurgitation, Tricuspid MDM in ASD, PSM in TR and VSD.

⇨ **Usually absent at cardiac apex:** ESM in pulmonary regurgitation, EDM in pulmonary regurgitation.

Murmurs at tricuspid area

⇨ **Only tricuspid area:** MDM in tricuspid stenosis, Tricuspid regurgitation(mild).

⇨ **Can be heard at tricuspid area:** AS, PS, AR, MR, VSD.

⇨ **Usually absent at tricuspid area:** MDM in mitral stenosis.

Murmurs at left 2nd ICS (pulmonary area)

⇨ **Best at pulmonary area:** PS, ASD flow murmur at pulmonary valve level, PR, PDA, VSD.

⇨ **Usually absent at pulmonary area:** Mitral stenosis MDM, Tricuspid stenosis MDM.

Murmurs at right 2nd ICS (aortic area)

⇨ **Best at aortic area:** Aortic root AR, AS(valvular), sclerosed aortic valve.

⇨ **Rarely at aortic area:** SM of pulmonary stenosis.

⇨ **Never at aortic area:** Mitral stenosis.

Murmurs at left 3rd ICS (Erb's area) near sternal border

⇨ **Best heard:** VSD (MC), EDM in aortic regurgitation, PS (infundibular), ESM in aortic stenosis.

⇨ **Can be heard sometimes:** PS (valvular), MR.

⇨ **Usually absent:** Mitral stenosis MDM.

Length/Duration

The length or duration of the murmur correlates directly to the severity of the lesion especially in stenotic lesions like MS, TS, PS or AS where it indicates the length of time of the pressure difference between two cardiac chambers.

Severity of regurgitant lesions producing pansystolic murmurs (PSM) like MR, TR or VSD may not be related to their length because even the mildest of these lesions may have PSM right from the beginning. However, whenever we hear a PSM, we should make it a habit to focus on the last 1/4th part of the murmur to see whether the murmur merges or ends before S2. If it ends before S2, it is an ejection murmur and not a PSM.

EDM of AR may sometimes have a direct correlation between the length and severity, but not as accurate as seen in stenotic lesions described above.

However, before correlating the length and severity of EDM of AR, we should consider the other associated conditions like CCF or acute onset AR which would produce a very short EDM despite severe AR.

Even conditions like hyperdynamic circulation or CCF can alter the relation between length and severity of lesions in stenotic lesions.

Grade or loudness of the murmur

Grade of the murmur is decided as per the Freeman and Levine grading system.

Diastolic murmurs irrespective of the grade are always organic or pathological.

Systolic murmurs are considered pathological or organic, once it reaches grade 4.

The loudness or intensity of the murmur relates directly to the severity of the turbulence.

↑loudness of the murmur	↓loudness of the murmur
↑flow velocity, e.g.; a small VSD.	↓flow velocity, e.g.; a large ASD.
Hyperdynamic states.	Hypodynamic states with ↓CO.
Thin and lean people.	Obese people, pleural effusion, pericardial effusion, COPD.

Grades of murmurs

- ⇨ **Grade I:** A very faint murmur requiring great concentration and effort to be heard.
- ⇨ **Grade II:** Easily heard
- ⇨ **Grade III:** Loud without thrill
- ⇨ **Grade IV:** Loud with thrill
- ⇨ **Grade V:** Murmur can be easily heard if the stethoscope is lightly applied to the chest
- ⇨ **Grade VI:** Murmur can be easily heard even if the stethoscope is lifted 1-1.5 cm above the chest wall.

Pitch of the murmur

Regurgitant murmurs ⇨ **high pitched.**

Stenotic murmurs ⇨ **low pitched.**

High pitched murmurs ⇨ called **BLOWING** murmurs.

Very clear pitch murmur with fundamental tones ⇨ **cooing/seagull** murmurs.

High pitch, high frequency murmurs ⇨ > 300 cps⇨ AR, MR (high pressure difference murmurs).

Medium pitch, medium frequency murmurs ⇨ 125-300 cps⇨ Flow murmurs, AS, PS, VSD, Innocent murmurs (high pressure difference murmurs).

Low pitch, low frequency murmurs ⇨ 25-125 cps⇨ TS, MS (low pressure difference murmurs).

Shape/configuration of the murmur

Shape of the murmur can be:

⇨ Crescendo: murmur keeps on ↑ in intensity, e.g.; ESM in AS.

⇨ Crescendo-decrescendo: progressive ↑ followed by progressive ↓ in intensity, e.g.; SM in AS due to systolic gradient changes between LV and aorta during ejection.

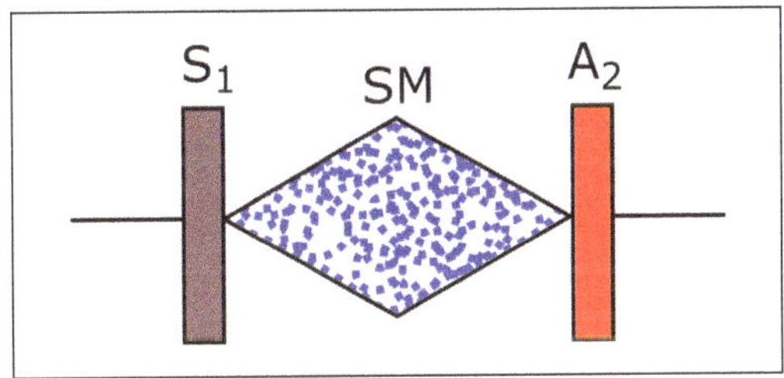

Fig. 14.4: SM of AS.

⇨ Decrescendo: murmur keeps on ↓ in intensity, e.g.; EDM in AR due to continuous ↓ in diastolic pressure gradient between aorta and LV.

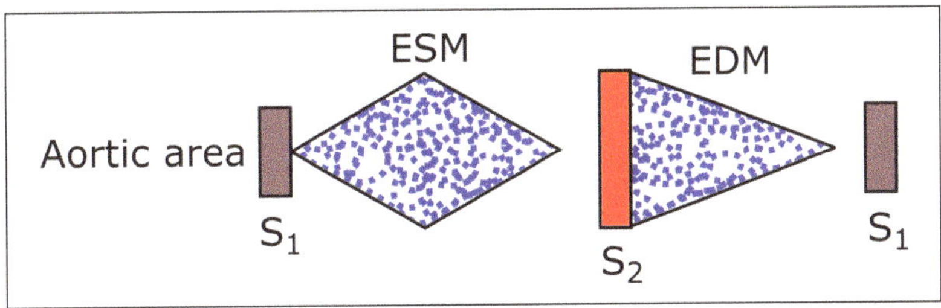

Fig. 14.5: EDM of acute AR.

- Plateau: constant intensity of the murmur, e.g.; PSM in MR due to maintenance of a constant and large pressure difference between the LV and LA.

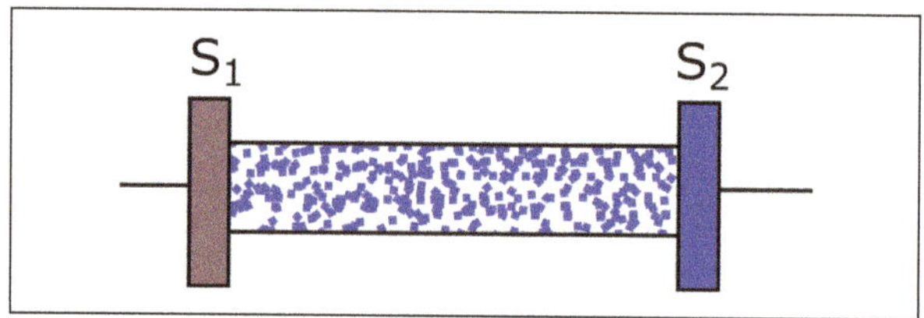

Fig. 14.6: PSM of MR.

Radiation to other site

- Radiation of the murmur is determined by its loudness, the direction of the blood flow and the condition of the chest wall.
- Radiation of the murmur can occur by means of the anatomic continuity as in AS where the SM is transmitted to the carotids or in MR where the PSM radiates to the axilla/back in anterior mitral leaflet (AML) involvement or to the base in posterior mitral leaflet (PML) involvement.
- Loud murmurs radiate widely whereas soft murmurs are usually restricted to the area where they originate.
- High frequency vibrations: (1) travels proximally to the site of its origin, e.g.; high frequency murmur of AS audible best at the apex (2) travels poorly through the chest wall (3) not associated with any thrill.
- Low frequency vibrations: (1) travels distally, e.g.; AS murmur harsh component usually is heard at the base and carotids (2) travels better through the chest wall (3) usually associated with a thrill.

Dynamic auscultation

Dynamic auscultation is a technique which is used to make heart sounds and murmurs prominent by means of physical maneuvers or drugs or positions/postures.

Commonly used procedures for dynamic auscultation are:

- Respiration
- Posture
- Exercise like sustained hand grip
- Valsalva and Muller maneuvers
- Arterial occlusion
- Changes in the cardiac cycle length by means of VPCs or Afib or Heart blocks
- Drugs like amyl nitrate, phenylephrine, etc.

Respiration

With Inspiration ⇨ ↓intrathoracic pressure ⇨ ↑RV venous return ⇨ ↑RV ejection time and RV stroke volume ⇨ ↑ pulmonary hangout interval > 80 msec.

Another scenario with Inspiration ⇨ ↓intrathoracic pressure⇨ ↑RV venous return ⇨ pulmonary pooling of blood ⇨ ↓ return to LV ⇨ ↓ LV ejection time and stroke volume ⇨ ↓ aortic hangout interval > 30 msec.

The expiratory events are just opposite to the inspiratory events.

Usually right-sided sounds/murmurs are louder on inspiration (except pulmonary ejection click which ↓ on inspiration) and left sided sounds/murmurs are louder on expiration.

Respiratory effects on cardiac sounds/murmurs:

Inspiration ⇨ Accentuated or ↑ OS (tricuspid), RVS3, RVS4, widened S2 split, increased pulmonary vascular ejection sound, ↑TR, MVP click louder and earlier (closer to S1 or S1-SC interval ↓), PR, TS, moderate PS.

Expiration⇨ Accentuated or ↑ OS(mitral), LVS3, LVS4, vascular aortic click, valvular pulmonary click, narrowed S2 split, MS, AR, VSD, pericardial rub.

> **NOTE**
>
> Since aortic diastolic pressure is always > LVEDP, the aortic valvular click does not change with respiration and so does the PSM of MR.

Posture

(1) Rapid standing from supine posture

↓venous return ⇨ ↓stroke volume⇨ reflex increases the HR and SVR immediately.

SPLITTING reduces, but truly fixed and split S2 remains unchanged.

Changes in cardiac sounds/murmurs with standing:

- ⇨ ↓RVS3, RVS4, LVS3, LVS4, narrowed S2 split
- ⇨ ↓SM of Semilunar valve stenosis (PS, AS), AV regurgitation murmurs (MR, TR), VSD, most of the functional systolic murmurs (due to ↓ SV)
- ⇨ Loud and early mid systolic click of MVP (due to ↓LVEDV)
- ⇨ ↑SM of HOCM (due to rise in the obstructive pressure gradient)

(2) Rapid supine from standing posture or rapid passive leg raising

↑venous return ⇨ sequential ↑ in RVEDV and then LVEDV ⇨ ↑stroke volume (both RV and LV) ⇨ ↑LV dimension after a few cardiac cycles ⇨ ↑ejection velocities.

Changes in cardiac sounds/murmurs with supine or rapid passive leg raising:

⇨ **Changes are opposite to what we saw in rapid standing from the supine posture described above.**

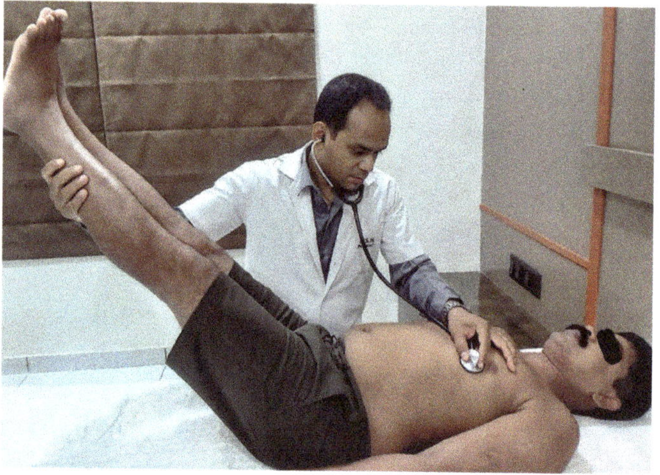

Fig. 14.7: Passive leg raising.

(3) Rapid squatting from standing posture

↑venous return⇨ ↑preload⇨ ↑SV ⇨ ↑arterial pressure with reflex bradycardia.

Also, rapid squatting⇨ kinking of bilateral femoral arteries⇨ ↑afterload due to ↑ systemic peripheral vascular resistance.

Changes in cardiac sounds/murmurs with rapid squatting:

⇨ ↑RVS3, RVS4, LVS3, LVS4 (all because of ↑SV)

⇨ ↑SM of AS, PS.

⇨ ↑DM of MS due to ↑preload leading to augmented diastolic flow across the MV

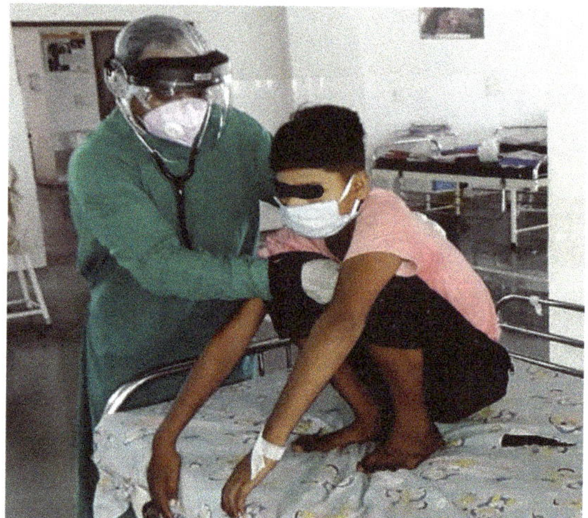

Fig. 14.8: Squatting posture.

⇨ ↑DM of AR, PSM of MR and SM of VSD due to ↑systemic peripheral vascular resistance and raised arterial pressure which causes ↑aortic reflux, ↑MR volume and ↑L→R shunting respectively.

⇨ ↓SM of HOCM due to ↑LV size and ↓LVOT obstruction.

⇨ Soft and delayed mid systolic click of MVP.

(4) Left lateral decubitus position (LLDP)

This position brings the heart closer to the chest wall and also leads to a slight ↑ in HR.

Changes in cardiac sounds/murmurs with LLDP:

⇨ ↑S1 (due to closeness of heart to the chest wall), LVS3, LVS4

⇨ ↑PreSM of AR (Austin Flint), SM of MR, MDM of MS

⇨ Loud and early Mid systolic click of MVP

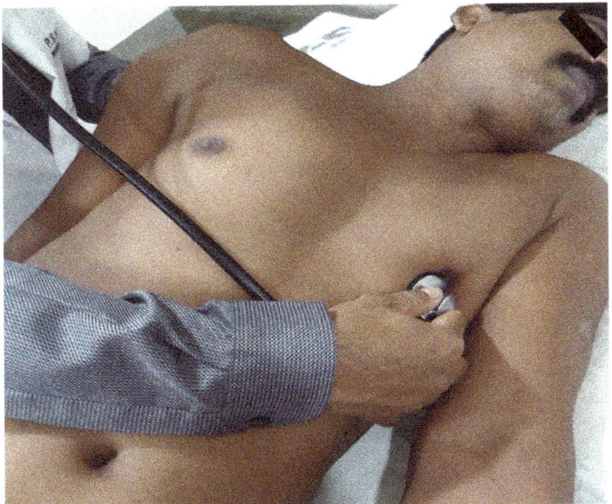

Fig. 14.9: Left lateral decubitus position.

(5) Sitting and leaning forward

This position brings the base of the heart close to the chest wall.

Changes in cardiac sounds/murmurs with leaning forward position:

⇨ ↑AR and PR diastolic murmurs

⇨ More clearer S2 split

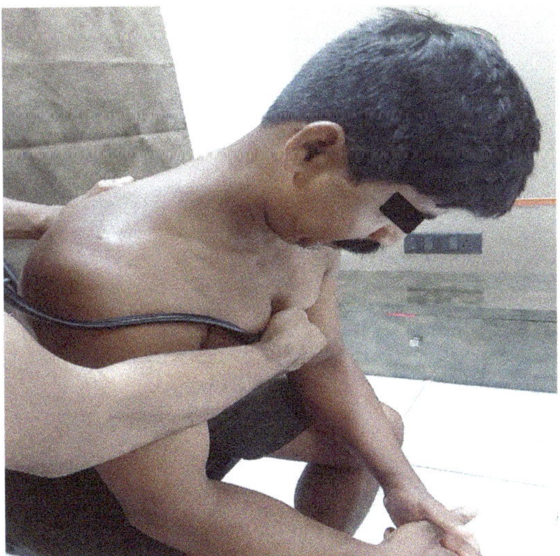

Fig. 14.10: Sitting and leaning forward.

(6) Knee-chest/Knee-elbow position

Better audibility of pericardial rub.

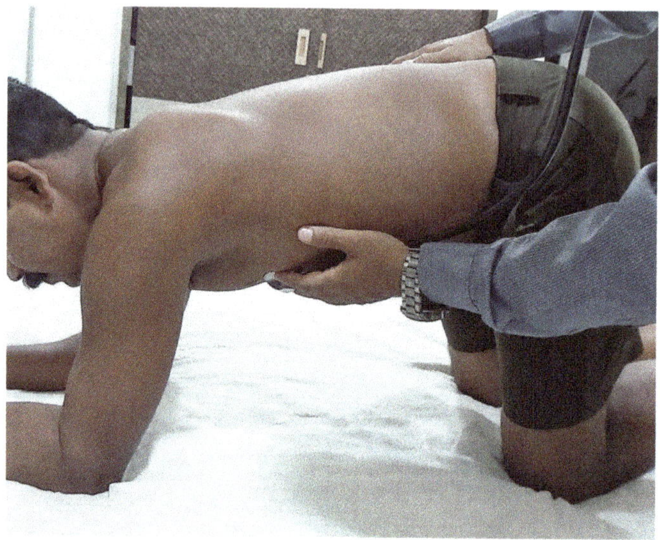

Fig. 14.11: Knee-elbow position.

Exercise

Sustained handgrip

Simply ask the patient to make a tight fist and hold it for 30 seconds.

This causes an ↑ in the HR, SVR, LV volume, LV filling pressure, CO, and blood pressure.

Done in supine posture and be careful with patients having IHD or hypertension or arrhythmias.

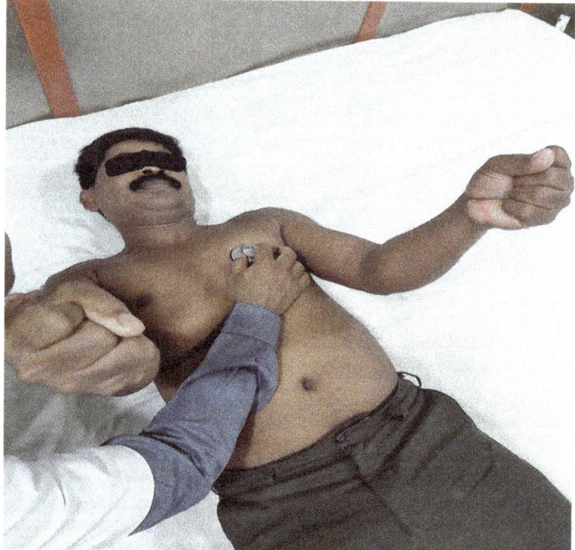

Fig. 14.12: Sustained handgrip.

Changes in cardiac sounds/murmurs with sustained handgrip:

- ⇨ Accentuated LVS3, LVS4
- ⇨ Loud MDM of MS due to ↑diastolic flow across the MV
- ⇨ ↑AR murmur (DM), SM of MR, murmur of VSD due to raised SVR
- ⇨ The SM of HOCM ↓
- ⇨ Soft and late mid systolic click of MVP

Valsalva maneuver

Discovered in 1704, where the patient used to blow with the nose and mouth closed to expel the pus from the middle ear.

At the bedside, this can be done by asking the patient to take a deep breath and then do a forceful expiration against a closed glottis for about 15 seconds.

We can place our hand on the patient's abdomen which would provide a pressure against which the patient has to blow and it also helps us to check for the extent and duration of the straining effort.

Phases of Valsalva maneuver:

- ⇨ **Phase I:** ↑intrathoracic pressure leads to rise in arterial pressure, ↑LV output and ↓HR. This phase is of 1-3 seconds duration.
- ⇨ **Phase II (strain phase):** ↓SV and venous return leading to a fall in BP and pulse pressure with reflex ↑ in HR.
- ⇨ **Phase III (release phase):** End of strain→↑venous return→with a ↓ in arterial pressure transiently. This phase lasts for 1-3 seconds.
- ⇨ **Phase IV:** Pooling of venous blood leading to ↑CO leading to ↑BP, wide pulse pressure and reflex ↓ in HR.

Phases I and III are undetectable at bedside.

Be careful while doing it in IHD patients as this maneuver ↓ the coronary blood supply.

Changes in cardiac sounds/murmurs with Valsalva maneuver:

Strain phase

- ⇨ Narrowed split of S2, ↓S3 and S4
- ⇨ ↑MVP and HOCM
- ⇨ ↓MS, AS, PS, AR, MR, PDA, VSD

Release phase

Exactly opposite changes occur compared to strain phase.

Mostly associated with ↑ in right sided murmurs due to ↑ venous return.

Valsalva maneuver can help us differentiate right sided SM from left sided ones.

On release of the Valsalva maneuver, the right sided murmurs usually return to their baseline intensity within 2-3 cardiac cycles whereas the left sided murmur takes a minimum of 5-10 cardiac cycles.

Muller maneuver

Reverse of Valsalva.

Patient inspires with the nose and mouth closed, for approximately 10-12 seconds.

It splits the S2 wide and makes the right sided murmurs prominent.

Arterial occlusion

When both the brachial arteries are transiently compressed externally by means of BP cuffs which are inflated 20-40 mmHg above the SBP for 20 seconds, the murmurs of MR, AR, and VSD are made prominent.

Ventricular premature contractions (VPC) or Atrial fibrillation(AF)

Following a VPC, there is a compensatory pause or with the longer cycle of atrial fibrillation, the ventricular function is augmented due to ↑ EDV and post extrasystolic potentiation of contraction leading to elevation of arterial pressure.

Changes in cardiac sounds/murmurs with VPC or AF:

⇨ Variable S1 due to AF

⇨ Accentuation of the SM of AS and PS

⇨ Prominent DM in AR (due to increased arterial pressure)

⇨ Prominent SM in HOCM (Brokenbrough Braunwald sign)

⇨ Soft and late mid systolic click of MVP

Drugs for dynamic auscultation

(1) Amyl nitrate

Administered by inhalation over 3-5 breaths over 10-12 seconds ⇨ ↓SVR ⇨ vasodilatation ⇨ ↓BP over the first 30 seconds.

After 30 seconds ⇨ ↓LV size ⇨ reflex tachycardia ⇨ ↑LV ejection or CO.

Changes in cardiac sounds/murmurs with amyl nitrate:

⇨ Augmentation of S1 and S3

⇨ ↑OS

⇨ ↓A2-OS interval

⇨ ↓A2

⇨ ↑SM of AS, PS, TR, HOCM (↑CO)

⇨ ↑murmurs of MS, TS, PR

⇨ Early and soft mid systolic click of MVP (due to small LV size and better LV ejection)

⇨ ↓DM in AR, ↓SM in TOF

⇨ MR induced S3 is ↓ due to ↓SVR

⇨ SEM of TOF is ↓ due to ↓BP, ↑ R→L shunt, ↓ RVOT blood flow

(2) Methoxamine and phenylephrine

Causes ↑ BP, reflex bradycardia, ↓cardiac contraction, ↓CO.

Phenylephrine is preferred due to its shorter action duration.

Both drugs are used cautiously in patients of CCF and hypertension.

Changes in cardiac sounds/murmurs with methoxamine and phenylephrine:

⇨ ↓S1

⇨ Loud A2

⇨ ↑A2-OS interval

⇨ ↑murmur of AR (both DM+Austin Flint murmur), MR, VSD, TOF, PDA (all because of raised arterial pressure)

⇨ ↓SM of HOCM and delayed MVP (due to ↑LV size)

⇨ ↓ESM in AS and DM of MS (due to ↓CO)

Cardiac murmurs that can be distinguished using dynamic maneuvers

Amyl nitrate

⇨ SM of TR↑ and MR↓

⇨ SM of AS↑ and MR↓

⇨ SM of PS↑ and VSD↓

⇨ SM of PS↑ and TOF↓

⇨ DM of AR (Austin Flint murmur)↓ and MS↑

⇨ EDM of PR↑ and AR↓

Respiration

⇨ SM of TR↑ and MR no change (INSPIRATION)

⇨ DM of MS↑ with expiration and DM of TS↑ with inspiration

⇨ EC of PS (valvular)↑ with expiration and ↓ with inspiration

Squatting

⇨ SM of HOCM↓and AS↑

Post-VPCs

⇨ SM of AS↑ and MR doesn't change

PATHOLOGIC MURMURS

There are some parameters which when present indicates that the murmur is not innocent or physiological, but pathological.

(1) Diastolic and continuous murmurs are always pathological.

(2) Murmurs with grade ≥ 4/6.

(3) Murmurs that are clearly radiating to other areas.

(4) Murmurs associated with thrills.

(5) Murmurs associated with cyanosis.

(6) Murmurs associated with abnormal cardiac rhythm.

(7) Pansystolic murmurs (PSM).

(8) Murmurs associated with abnormal S2, i.e.; paradoxical split S2 or widely split S2 or single S2.

References

- Bonow RO, Carabello BA, Chatterjee K, de Leon AC Jr, Faxon DP, Freed MD, Gaasch WH, Lytle BW, Nishimura RA, O'Gara PT, O'Rourke RA, Otto CM, Shah PM, Shanewise JS. ACC/AHA 2006 guidelines for the management of patients with valvular heart disease: a report of the American College of Cardiology/American Heart Association Task Force on Practice Guidelines (Writing Committee to Develop Guidelines for the Management of Patients With Valvular Heart Disease). Circulation. 2006;114:e84 - e231. DOI: 10.1161/CIRCULATIONAHA.106.176857.
- Synopsis of cardiac physical diagnosis; 2nd edition; Jonathan Abrams.
- Clinical examination in cardiology; 2nd edition; B N VIJAY RAGHAWA RAO.
- The art and science of cardiac physical examination; 2nd edition; Narasimhan Ranganathan.
- Clinical methods in cardiology by B Soma Raju.
- Martin, Nicole, and Leonard S. Lilly. "The cardiac cycle: Mechanisms of heart sounds and murmurs." Pathophysiology of Heart Disease: A Collaboration Project of Medical Students and Faculty 4th ed (2007): 29-45.
- Harrison's Principles of Internal medicine, 18th edition, CHAPTER e13 Approach to the Patient With a Heart Murmur.
- JIACM 2012; 13(4): 299-302;M Chaturvedi, A Pandey, Ankesh Kumar, Ankur Pandey;Dynamic auscultation - A lost art which needs to be revived.
- J Pediatr (Rio J) 2003;79 Suppl 1:S87-S96: heart defects, congenital, heart auscultation, heartMurmurs; Assessment of heart murmurs in childhood by Maria Elisabeth B.A. Kobinger.

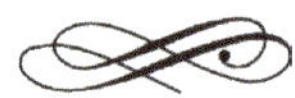

CHAPTER 15 Systolic Murmurs

Murmur starts at or just after S1, but ending before S2 (this can be checked by palpating the carotid upstroke and apex thrust that occurs immediately after S1, discussed in earlier chapters).

Systolic murmurs are further sub-classified as:-

⇨ **Early systolic (ESM):** Starts with S1 and ending before mid-systole. Usually decrescendo in configuration.

⇨ **Mid systolic (MSM):** Starts after S1 and and ending before respective A2 or P2, i.e.; S2. Also called **ejection systolic murmur**. Has crescendo-decrescendo type of configuration (diamond shaped murmurs) as these are produced due to ejection from the ventricles to their respective greater arteries.

Thus, the series of events are S1→isovolumetric contraction→ ejection systolic murmur→hangout interval→S2.

↑ejection→murmur↑.

↓ejection→murmur↓.

⇨ **Late systolic (LSM):** Usually begins after ejection and terminates at or before S2. High pitched murmurs.

⇨ **Pan- or Holosystolic (PSM):** Occupies the whole period from S1 to S2 due to a wide difference in pressures between two cardiac chambers like LV→LA or LV→RV.

EARLY SYSTOLIC MURMUR (ESM)

(1) **Small muscular VSD**→ Shunting occurs only during the early part of systole because with cardiac contraction, the small defect is sealed off during the later part of contraction and the flow is terminated.

(2) **Large nonrestrictive VSD with increased PVR**→ The shunting of blood in the late systolic period is halted due to raised PVR.

(3) **Severe MR of acute onset**→ Can occur after MI leading to papillary muscle rupture, SABE, trauma leading to mitral valve damage, myxomatous degeneration leading to chordae rupture, etc.

(4) **TR with normal systolic pressure of RV**→ Cardiac surgeries, trauma, drug abusers, infarction of RV, carcinoid disease.

(5) **Childhood innocent murmurs**.

MIDSYSTOLIC EJECTION MURMURS

Can be caused by:

⇨ Obstruction to the ventricular outflow tract

- AS, PS, HOCM, TOF, Sub- and Supra-valvular aortic stenosis

⇨ ↑flow across the semilunar valves (functional)

- ASD, VSD,

⇨ Dilated root of aorta or pulmonary trunk (functional)

⇨ Diseased semilunar valves

- Aortic sclerosis

⇨ Innocent murmurs (functional)

Etiologies of LVOT obstruction

At the valvular level: Rheumatic AS, bicuspid aortic valve, unicuspid aortic valve, myxoid degeneration, severe calcification, Fabry's disease, IE.

At the supravalvular level: Hourglass congenital abnormality of aorta, dissection of the aorta, discrete membranous congenital abnormality of aorta, Rubella infection.

At the subvalvular level: HOCM, tunnel and discrete membranous types of aortic stenosis.

Etiologies of RVOT obstruction

At the valvular level: Single commissure of PV, domed PV, bicuspid PV, PV hypoplasia, PV dysplasia, Rheumatic degeneration, carcinoid syndrome.

At the supravalvular level: Congenital stenosis, main pulmonary trunk stenosis, peripheral pulmonary stenosis (right and left), neoplastic compression, Rubella.

At the subvalvular level: Congenital stenosis, stenosis at the infundibulum, tumor, fibromuscular tissue below the valve.

VALVULAR AORTIC STENOSIS

The murmur of valvular AS is a diamond shaped, mixed frequency ejection systolic murmur, consisting of both high frequency and low frequency sounds, and has a rough quality. Usually not more than 3/6 grade.

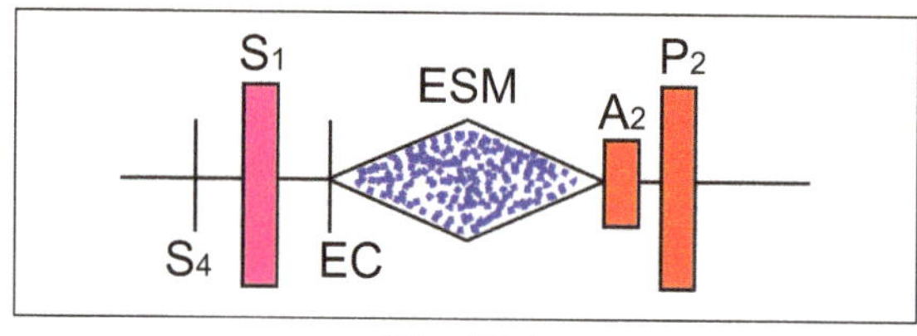

Fig. 15.1

Area of best audibility

⇨ Rough component/low frequency - Aortic area and radiates to the carotids (especially right side)

⇨ High frequencies – Apex (may sometimes be confused with murmur of MR which is called **Gallavardin phenomenon**, but doesn't radiate to the axilla like MR murmur).

The murmur of AS also ends before S2, unlike MR murmur which may go upto S2.

> **NOTE**
>
> (1) Subvalvular AS ⇨ Left sternal border without carotid involvement.
>
> (2) Supravalvular AS ⇨ Only carotid murmur with/without aortic area involvement.
>
> (3) AS murmur only at the apex ⇨ Emphysema with calcified aortic valves where only the apical part of the heart is in contact with the chest wall.

Dynamic auscultation of AS murmur

Murmur↑	Murmur↓
Squatting	Valsalva phase II
Post VPCs	Sustained handgrip
Valsalva phase III	∝ adrenergic agonist drugs
Passive leg raising	
Amyl nitrate administration	

Factors determining the severity of AS

(1) Longer the murmur, more severe the AS.

Duration of the murmur indicates how long the pressure difference across the valve is sustained, as with severe AS the LV has to contract for a longer time to eject the desired amount of blood (**sustained apical impulse**).

(2) Early peaking murmur - mild AS.

Late peaking murmur - severe AS.

(3) **Delayed upstroke of carotid pulse** or slow rising pulse - severe AS (most accurate sign clinically).

(4) Paradoxical splitting of S2 - severe AS.

(5) Intensity of the murmur sometimes may indicate the severity of the AS (not reliable).

Carotid pulse in valvular AS

⇨ pulsus parvus et tardus

⇨ volume is small

⇨ thrill which is palpable

⇨ non-palpable prominent anacrotic notch

However, conditions with ↑CO can cause OVERESTIMATION of the severity of AS like:

⇨ Hyperdynamic circulatory states, e.g.; anaemia, thyrotoxicosis, pregnancy, etc.

⇨ Additional PDA or AR

⇨ ↑HR

UNDERESTIMATION of the severity of AS

⇨ CCF

⇨ MS, TS (proximal obstruction)

⇨ IHD

⇨ Hypothyroidism

⇨ MR, VSD (proximal shunt and regurgitation)

⇨ Cardiac arrhythmias

Importance of ejection click in AS

⇨ It indicates that the obstruction is at the level of the aortic valve proper

⇨ The aortic valves are pliable

⇨ The AS is of milder grade.

A2 in valvular AS

⇨ The A2 is delayed and is of low intensity in severe AS

⇨ Even with paradoxical split of S2, the murmur ends before A2

⇨ In very severe AS, the A2 may even be absent.

Many patients with valvular AS can have concomitant AR which have its own significance.

Presence of AR in a patient who already has AS indicates that

⇨ the obstruction is either fixed valvular or it is subvalvular in location

⇨ the SM is mostly due to the AS or an associated VSD.

A new onset AR in a patient who already has AS indicates a high probability of Infective endocarditis.

Timing of the murmur

Early onset ejection with early onset murmur:

- ⇨ Severe AR (due to low aortic diastolic pressure)
- ⇨ Hyperdynamic circulation

Late onset ejection with late onset murmur:

- ⇨ Severe LV dysfunction (due to high aortic diastolic pressure).

SUPRAVALVULAR AORTIC STENOSIS

Supravalvular aortic stenosis is associated with a SM which can be differentiated from the ejection systolic murmur of valvular aortic stenosis by the facts that:

- ⇨ the SM radiates to both the carotids and can be heard best only at the right 2nd ICS (aortic area).
- ⇨ absence of Gallavardin phenomenon
- ⇨ no ejection click (since it is not valvular)
- ⇨ the blood jet in supravalvular aortic stenosis is directed more towards the right brachiocephalic artery due to which, right brachial and carotid pulse amplitude is > left brachial and carotid pulse amplitude.

Usually discovered in childhood itself due to associated mental retardation and Elfin facies (William's syndrome).

SUB VALVULAR AORTIC STENOSIS

May be fixed (discrete membranous and tunnel type stenosis) or dynamic(HOCM).

No ejection click.

Chest X-ray may not show dilatation of ascending aorta.

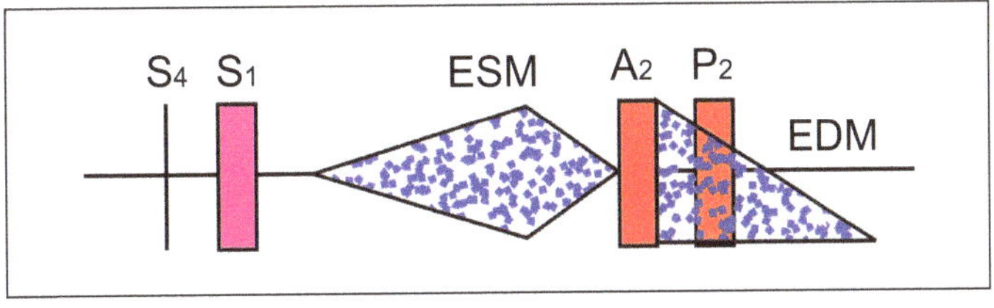

Fig. 15.2

(1) Hypertrophic cardiomyopathy

Also called Idiopathic hypertrophic subaortic stenosis (IHSS).

Hallmark - massive asymmetric thickening of the interventricular septum with displacement of the AML and the anterolateral papillary muscle.

Blood outflow from the LV is obstructed during mid- to late systole.

The ejection of blood from the LV is so rapid in HOCM that by the end of mid systole, the LV is emptied by 85-90% and shrinks in size.

In addition, there is systolic anterior motion (SAM) of the AML that touches the IVS in mid- to late systole due to Venturi effect of rapid blood ejection and causes dynamic obstruction to the LV outflow.

The LV compliance is ↓ due to hypertrophied and stiff LV with ↑ filling pressure and dilated LA.

30 - 50% patients show MR which corresponds to SAM on echocardiography.

Symptoms

- ⇨ Breathlessness on exertion: ↑ LV filling pressures
- ⇨ Chest pain: ↑ myocardial O_2 demand of the hypertrophied LV
- ⇨ Syncope: LVOT obstruction
- ⇨ Sudden death: severe ventricular arrhythmias

Clinical findings

JVP: Large a waves due to ventricular noncompliance and significant atrial contraction.

Carotid pulse: Rapid upstroke→midsystolic dip→late systolic wave.

Carotid thrill is common in HOCM in contrast to valvular AS.

LV impulse: Heaving in late systole in left lower sternal border in lateral decubitus associated with a thrill commonly which indicates LVOT obstruction.

Heart sounds

- ⇨ Loud S1
- ⇨ Paradoxically split S2, due to prolonged LV ejection due to obstruction leading to delayed A2
- ⇨ Occasional S3 due to noncompliant ventricles
- ⇨ S4 due to strong atrial contraction.

Murmur of HOCM

⇨ Crescendo-decrescendo SM with peak in late systole

⇨ Medium pitched (but higher than murmur of AS)

⇨ Best heard along the left lower sternal border

⇨ May radiate to base of neck but usually do not radiates to the carotids

⇨ The SM is longer when there is associated MR.

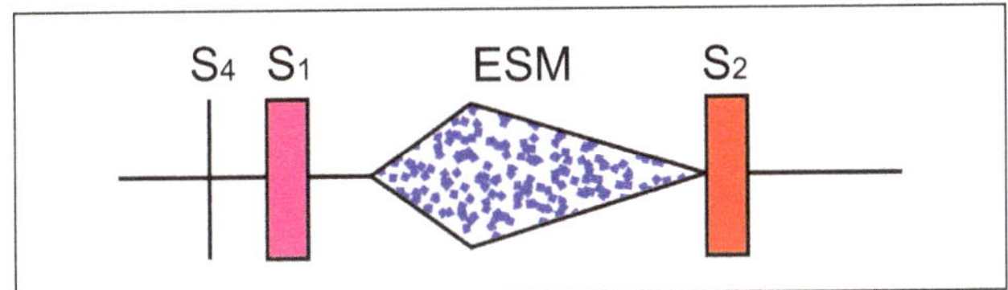

Fig. 15.3: Murmur of HOCM.

Factors that makes the SM louder

⇨ ↓ preload

⇨ ↓ afterload

⇨ ↑ contraction of LV

The reverse is true for factors that make the SM softer.

Dynamic auscultation in HOCM

↑ loudness of SM⇨ Valsalva phase II, standing, post VPCs, amyl nitrate.

↓ loudness of SM⇨ Supine posture, passive leg raising, squatting, sustained handgrip, ∝ adrenergic drugs.

(2) Discrete subaortic stenosis

Fixed obstruction due to fibrous web/fibromuscular tunnel.

SM similar to AS but, without a click.

No post stenotic dilatation of aorta on chest X-ray.

PULMONARY STENOSIS

Congenital causes→ MC cause of pulmonic stenosis.

Pulmonary stenosis can be at the level of

(1) Valve proper

(2) Subvalvular→ infundibular (10% of the total cases of RVOT obstruction), double chambered RV, tumor, thrombus

(3) Supravalvular→ congenital, rubella, neoplasm, thrombus.

The murmur of pulmonary valve stenosis is a harsh, ejection systolic murmur with a harsh crescendo-decrescendo quality that peaks in late systole. Usually 3/6 or greater in grade.

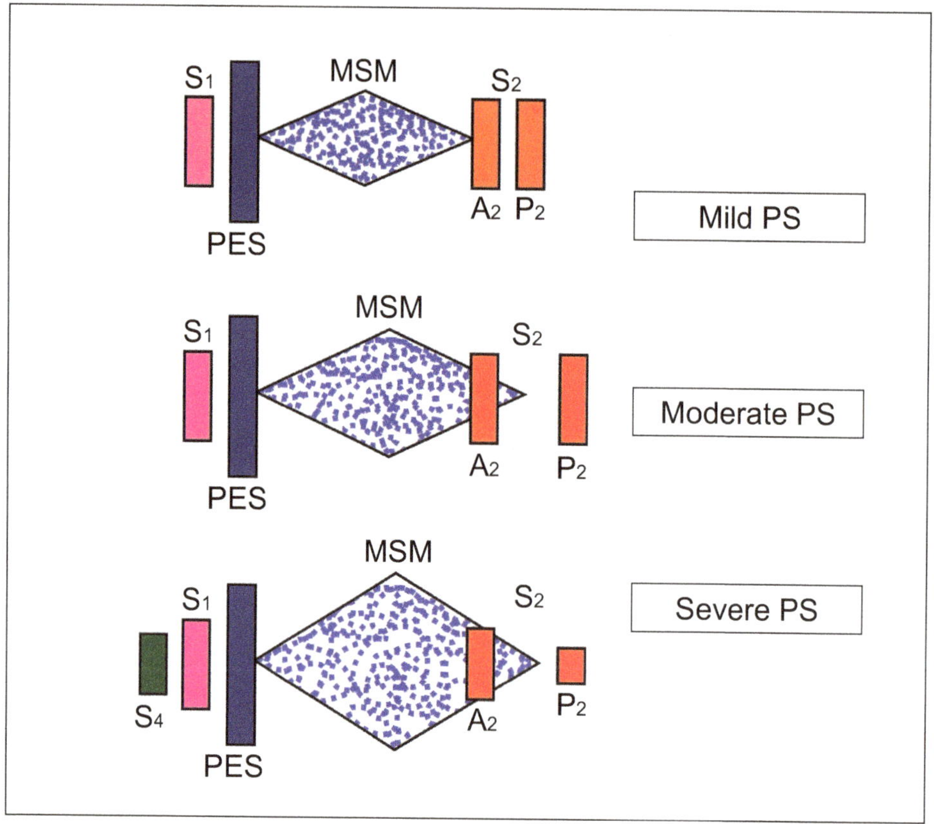

Fig. 15.4: Murmur of PS.

Site of best audibility

(1) Pulmonary valve stenosis ⇨ Pulmonary area with conduction to the left side of the neck. Sometimes can also be heard at the aortic area or the right 3rd ICS.

(2) Infundibular PS or double chambered RV ⇨ Erb's area or the left 4th ICS (with failure of conduction to left side in infundibular PS).

(3) Supravalvular PS ⇨ Infraclavicular

(4) Pulmonary stenosis with L-Transposition of great arteries (L-TGA) ⇨ Aortic area or the right 3rd ICS (since PA is posterior and to the right).

Distinguishing PS from VSD

	PS	VSD
S2	Wide split	Normal
Conduction to left side of the neck	Present	Absent
Accompanying features	Prominent a waves, parasternal heave, S4, ejection click	Nil

NOTE

Ejection click localizes the stenosis to the valve level. However, there are few conditions where the ejection click may be absent despite having a valvular PS like PV dysplasia, PV atresia, PS of very severe grade.

Distinguishing PS murmur from AS murmur

	AS	PS
Radiation	Widely radiates	Radiates less compared to AS murmur
Relation with inspiration	Does Not change	↑ with inspiration
Relation with S2	Goes upto A2	Goes upto P2 after extending from A2

Accessing the severity of PS

The severity of PS is indicated by its intensity, length and time to peak.

Increase in all these parameters are directly associated with the severity of the PS.

Hence, a loud, lengthy ejection murmur of PS which peaks very late in systole indicates a severe PS.

However, it is very important to understand that these parameters are inversely related to the severity of PS in TOF. This is because in TOF there is associated VSD which helps to shunt the blood from the RV to LV as the severity of the PS increases.

Associated features in PS

- S2→ Wide split with soft P2 component
- S4→ Indicates severe PS
- Dominant a wave in JVP
- Parasternal heave

Dynamic auscultation in valvular PS

↑ loudness of SM⇨ Valsalva phase III, post VPCs, amyl nitrate, passive leg raising

Syndromes associated with PS

⇨ Noonan syndrome

⇨ Rubella syndrome

Grading the severity of PS depending on the gradient across the stenosis

⇨ less than 50 mmHg: mild PS

⇨ 50 to 70 mmHg: moderate PS

⇨ more than 70 mmHg: severe PS

ATRIAL SEPTAL DEFECT (ASD)

ASD can also produce a SM due to ↑ flow across the RVOT.

This is more or less like a functional murmur only, but unlike functional murmurs the SM in ASD is associated with a wide fixed split S2.

The widely split and fixed S2 with a loud P2 in ASD helps differentiate it from the murmur of PS where the S2 is split but not fixed and also the P2 is not loud.

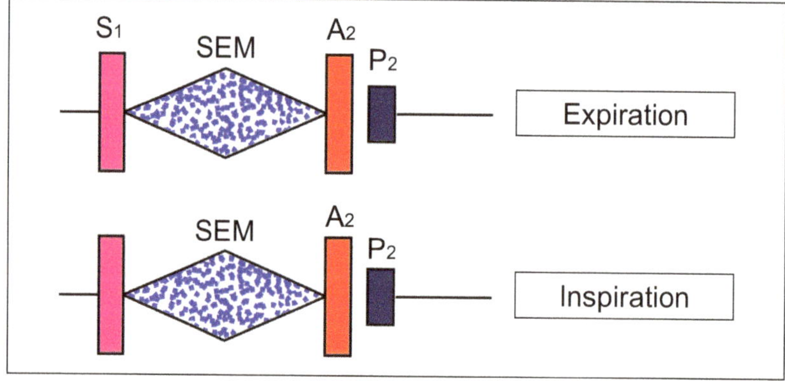

Fig. 15.5

TETRALOGY OF FALLOT (TOF)

TOF comprises of:

⇨ infundibular PS

⇨ VSD

⇨ overriding of aorta

⇨ RVH

In TOF:

⇨ mild PS: murmur occurs due to the VSD

⇨ moderate to severe PS: murmur occurs due to RVOT obstruction.

When the PS is mild in TOF

⇨ murmur is harsher with a crescendo-decrescendo nature and peaks late in systole.

⇨ this murmur is grade 4/6 or more usually.

⇨ the P2 is soft and delayed.

When the PS is severe in TOF

⇨ more blood is shifted across the VSD from RV to LV and thus the murmur peaks early in systole with an occasional aortic flow murmur audible.

⇨ the P2 is absent.

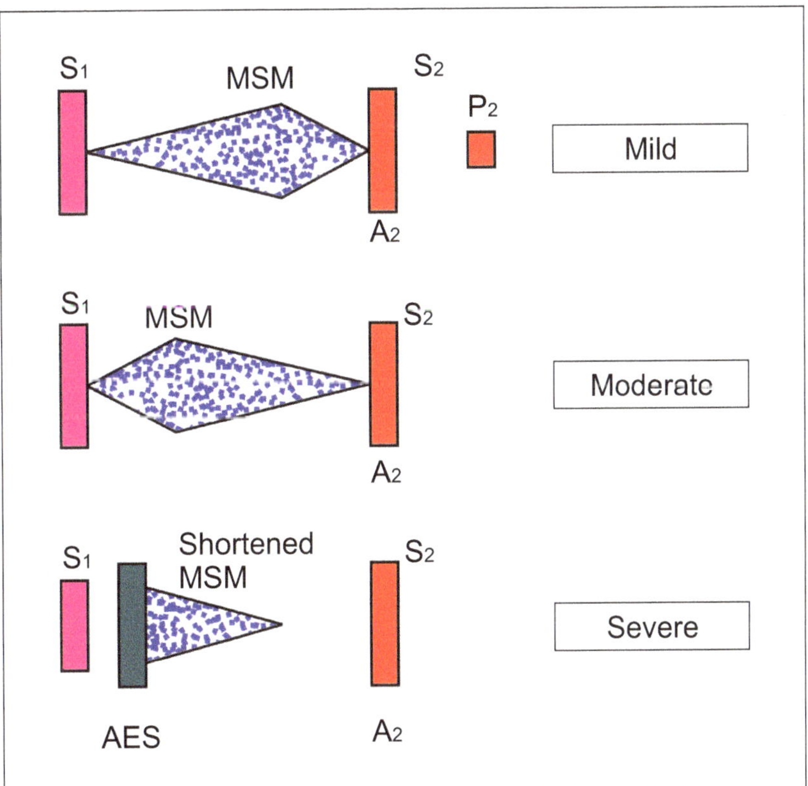

Fig. 15.6: Murmur of PS in TOF.

FUNCTIONAL EJECTION SYSTOLIC MURMURS

No underlying cardiac disease.

These are heard in healthy individuals.

Commonly found in children and some hyperdynamic circulatory states.

May disappear as the child grows.

Aggravated by anxiety and exertion.

Functional murmurs include

⇨ Still's murmur

⇨ ↑flow through the pulmonary root

⇨ murmurs due to hyperdynamic circulatory states

⇨ flow murmurs due to AR and PR

⇨ pulmonary branch murmur

⇨ supraclavicular murmur

⇨ murmur due to aortic sclerosis

⇨ murmur due to dilated aortic root or pulmonary artery trunk

(1) Still's murmur

→ MC innocent murmur of childhood

→ 75-85 % of school going children are affected

→ Commonly heard along the left sternal border at the Erb's area or the left 4th ICS.

→ Mid systolic, non radiating, low to medium pitched ejection murmur due to ↑ flow across a normal LVOT.

→ D/D includes small VSD, HOCM, discrete subaortic stenosis.

(2) ↑flow through pulmonary root/pulmonary ejection murmur

→ MC between the ages of 8-14 years

→ High pitched

→ Blowing quality

→ Better heard at left 2nd ICS (pulmonary area)

→ D/D includes ASD and PV stenosis

(3) Murmurs due to hyperdynamic circulatory states

→ These conditions cause an ↑ flow across the aorta leading to the functional murmur.

→ Includes conditions like hyperthyroidism, pregnancy, fever, anemia, AV fistula, etc.

(4) Flow murmurs due to AR and PR

→ AR and PR causes an ↑ in the SV that must pass through the ventricular outflow tracts.

→ These murmurs typically peak in mid systole

→ Medium pitched, crescendo-decrescendo

→ Do not radiate

→ Heard best at the aortic and pulmonary areas respectively.

→ Usually upto grades 3/6, but sometimes can be grade 4 also with a thrill in cases of very severe AR.

(5) Pulmonary branch murmur

→ Occurs mostly in premature and low birth weight babies

→ Right and left pulmonary branch hypoplasia is present

→ Pathological pulmonary branch stenosis - if there is persistence of the murmur > 6 months of age.

→ Best audible area - upper part of left sternum

→ Radiation - thorax, axilla and back.

(6) Supraclavicular murmur

→ Heard above the carotid arteries in the supraclavicular fossa.

→ Originates from the brachiocephalic artery

→ May be wrongly diagnosed as an organic systolic murmur

→ It disappears with hyperextension of the shoulders in the later part of the systole.

(7) Aortic sclerosis

→ Commonly seen in elderly above 50 years of age (50%).

→ Also called "50-50" murmur

→ There is thickening of the aortic valve with mild calcification occasionally as a result of which the valve does not open properly causing turbulence and the murmur.

→ **Ejection systolic murmur** in aortic sclerosis is softer than AS murmur, and is short with early systolic peaking.

→ **S2** is split normally

→ **A2** is usually normal, but may be loud sometimes

→ There is no associated fourth heart sound or LV hypertrophy, and the pulse is normal.

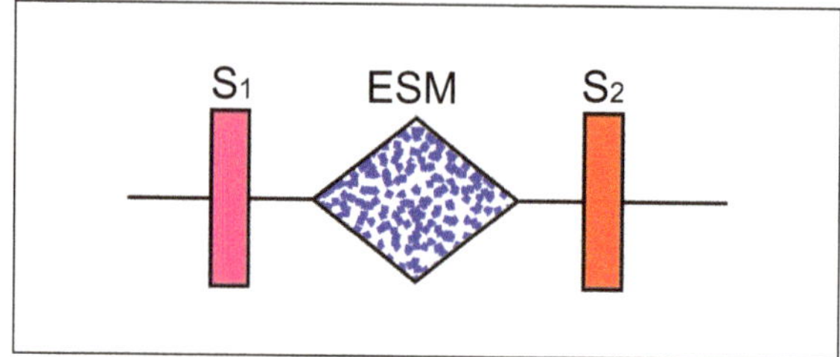

Fig. 15.7: Murmur of aortic sclerosis.

(8) Murmur due to aortic root dilatation (commonly due to sclerosis) or pulmonary artery trunk dilatation due to PAH.

MID SYSTOLIC MURMUR DUE TO IHD

This can occur due to damage to the papillary muscles leading to MR that causes the mid systolic murmur.

LATE SYSTOLIC MURMURS

May be caused by:

⇨ Mitral valve prolapse (MVP)/Tricuspid valve prolapse

⇨ Papillary dysfunction

Mitral valve prolapse (MVP)

→ Medium pitched

→ Crescendo in nature

→ Associated with non ejection click

→ Site of best audibility is apex

→ Does not radiate

→ Factors that ↓ the LV volume may make the murmur pansystolic with a honking or whooping quality (e.g.; sudden standing).

Dynamic auscultation in MVP

↑ loudness of murmur with early systolic click(click moves closer to S1: Valsalva phase II, sudden standing, amyl nitrate.

↓ loudness of murmur with delayed systolic click: Post VPCs, supine posture, passive leg raising, squatting, sustained handgrip, ∝ adrenergic drugs.

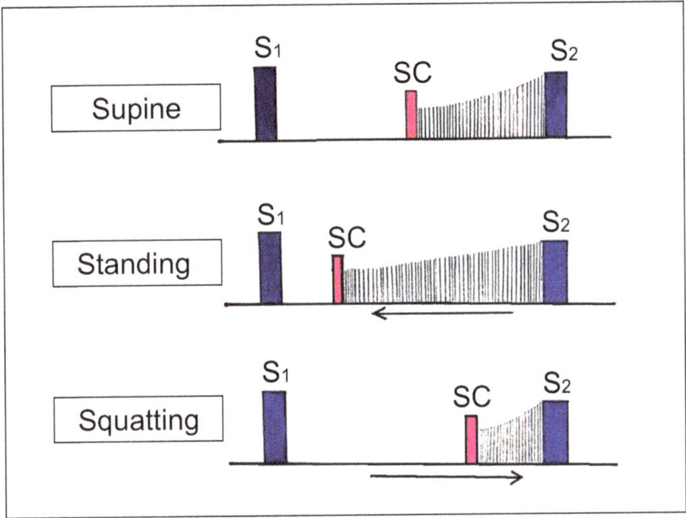

Fig. 15.8: Murmur of MVP.

PANSYSTOLIC MURMUR

The murmur occupies the whole period from S1 to S2.

PSM occurs when there is a wide pressure difference between two cardiac chambers which is maintained for a long period in cardiac cycle.

In cardiology, a PSM occurs only in 3 conditions:

⇨ MR - pressure difference maintained between LV and LA

⇨ TR - pressure difference maintained between RV and RA

⇨ VSD - pressure difference maintained between LV and RV

MITRAL REGURGITATION (MR)

The mitral valve apparatus consists of the mitral valve leaflets, annulus, chordae, the papillary muscles, and the LA and LV.

Abnormality of any of the above components leads to MR where blood regurgitates into the LA from LV under high pressure at the onset of the LV contraction and continues till the end of it.

Rheumatic heart disease is the MC cause of MR, leading to damage to the valve cusps and their retraction along with fusion of the commissures. The chordae tendineae also shortens and fuses together which can add a stenotic component to the regurgitation.

Causes of MR

⇨ Abnormalities of Mitral leaflets: RHD, MVP, IE.

⇨ Papillary damage: IHD, severely dilated LV (lateral displacement), fibrotic changes, etc.

⇨ Damage to the chordae tendineae: Trauma, IE, etc.

⇨ Mitral annular calcification.

Time of the murmur

⇨ PSM is the classical murmur in MR.

However, in acute MR, the normal LA has a normal compliance and cannot cope with the sudden increase in blood volume due to regurgitation from the LV. This leads to sudden rise of the LA pressure during systole leading to a murmur which is Early systolic in nature with a decrescendo contour and terminates before S2. The sudden rise in LA pressure leads to ↑ in pulmonary venous pressure that causes acute pulmonary edema.

With the passage of time, both LA and LV dilates.

The murmur of classical chronic MR is usually of grade 3/6 without any thrill.

Thrill in MR occurs with (1) damage to the chordae or (2) IE or (3) if AS or VSD is wrongly diagnosed as MR.

Causes of MR not producing PSM:

- Acute MR
- Papillary rupture
- MVP
- Very mild and negligible MR

Silent MR:

- Trivial MR (MC cause)
- MR in LV dysfunction (IHD or CCF)
- Periprosthetic MR
- IE
- Obesity
- COPD
- Large LA

Area of best audibility

⇨ Apex. Sometimes also heard at the left lower sternal border.

Murmur of MVP - left lower sternal border.

Character of the murmur

⇨ Rheumatic MR - soft and blowing

⇨ MR due to chordal rupture or IE - cooing nature or “seagull” quality

⇨ MR with flail leaflets - musical quality

⇨ MR due to MVP - honking and rasping with a harsh quality

Radiation of the murmur

⇨ Rheumatic MR radiating to the left axilla and back - AML damage leading to posteriorly directed blood jet

⇨ MR due to MVP radiating to the base (aortic area) - PML damage leading to an anteriorly and medially directed jet along the root of the aorta

⇨ MR in pediatric population - murmur at the left 2nd ICS due to jet directed towards the LAA which lies close to the PA.

Dynamic auscultation

⇨ Respiration: The murmur of MR remains unchanged with expiration.

⇨ Posture: MR murmur due to RHD ↓on standing.

MR due to MVP ↑on standing and ↓on lying down.

⇨ Valsalva: RHD MR - ↓.

MVP MR - ↑ during strain phase.

⇨ ∝ adrenergic drugs: MVP MR ↓.

Carotid pulse in MR

⇨ Sharp but pulse volume is reduced.

⇨ Water hammer pulse in severe MR.

⇨ Normal arterial pulse.

JVP

⇨ Prominent v waves due to functional TR due to PAH.

Apex beat

⇨ Hyperdynamic and displaced downward and outward.

⇨ Sometimes a diastolic outward thrust is felt indicative of a palpable S3.

Parasternal lift

⇨ Occurs due to the enlarged LA pushing on the anteriorly placed RV.

Cardiac sounds

- ⇨ Soft S1 (sometimes loud if associated MS present)
- ⇨ S2 - widely split with inspiration (only in severe cases)
- ⇨ S3 indicates large regurgitated volume and LV dysfunction
- ⇨ S4 if present, is always right sided in MR because the dilated LA is not able to contract and generate a left sided S4.
- ⇨ Mid diastolic murmur(MDM) is possible in severe MR due increased volume and rapid flow into the LV.

TRICUSPID REGURGITATION (TR)

The MC cause of TR is functional because of PAH leading to RV dilatation that in turn causes dilatation of the TV annulus (80%).

Causes of TR

- ⇨ Primary TR: RHD, IE, myxomatous degeneration, radiation, carcinoid syndrome, Ebstein's anomaly, MI.
- ⇨ Functional TR: Any cause of RV dilatation leading to TV annular dilatation like PAH, MI, etc.

Pathophysiology

The regurgitant volume depends on the RV systolic pressure and the area of the regurgitant orifice.

The RV CO is decreased and over the time there is dilation of RA and RV both. The JVP is raised.

There is 'ventricularization' of the waveforms of RA.

The murmur of TR

Area of best audibility

- ⇨ Left lower sternal border or tricuspid area (TA)
- ⇨ Murmur of Ebstein's anomaly: just lateral to the apex
- ⇨ Severe TR with RV enlargement: murmur best heard at the apex and sometimes confused with MR.

Time of the murmur

- ⇨ The murmur of typical TR is a high pitched, blowing, Pansystolic murmur (PSM) which indicates a sustained pressure difference between the RV and RA.

The duration and pitch of the murmur is directly related to the pressure rise in the RV.

However, in the absence of PAH, even an organic TR may produce a non PSM or short murmur, e.g.; RHD, TVP, carcinoid syndrome, IE, very mild TR, etc.

A PSM indicates an RVSP of minimum 70-72 mmHg.

Grade of the murmur

⇨ Usually < 3/6

⇨ No thrill.

⇨ Presence of thrill in TR should alert you regarding the presence of a VSD which is wrongly interpreted as TR.

Radiation of the murmur

⇨ Usually no radiation

⇨ In severe TR sometimes the jet may flow towards the SVC wherein the murmur may radiate to the neck.

Dynamic auscultation

⇨ ↑loudness of the murmur: Inspiration (Carvallo's sign) (due to increased filling during inspiration), post VPCs, amyl nitrate, passive leg raising.

⇨ ↓loudness of the murmur: Expiration, standing, straining phase of Valsalva.

The changes with respiration helps to distinguish murmur of TR from MR.

Parasternal impulse

⇨ Heaving: TR with PAH

⇨ Hyperdynamic: Organic TR without PAH

RVS3

⇨ Indicates rapid filling of a failing RV.

⇨ Indicates that there is no associated TS.

JVP

⇨ Prominent c-v waves

⇨ Rapid y descent (indicates no TS)

Diastolic murmur (DM) in TR

⇨ Sometimes when the TR volume is very large, it causes increased flow during the ventricular filling phase and may produce a diastolic murmur which is a sign of absent TS.

VENTRICULAR SEPTAL DEFECT (VSD)

In VSD, there is a hole or defect in the interventricular septum(IVS) that separates the LV and RV.

VSDs constitute 20% of all congenital heart diseases (CHD).

VSDs can occur as an isolated entity or may occur as a part of complex syndromes consisting of cTGA, TOF, truncus arteriosus, ASD, D-TGA, double outlet RV, etc.

Various syndromes associated with VSD are CHARGE syndrome, Trisomy 21, Edward's syndrome, etc.

Parts of the IVS

- ⇨ Inlet part: Smooth extension from tricuspid septal cusp to the tensor apparatus of tricuspid (also known as the AV canal septum).
- ⇨ Trabecular part: Separates the apical RV from LV. Also called the muscular septum.
- ⇨ Infundibular/Outlet part: Smooth region. The septal band separates this region from the trabeculated area of the RV.
- ⇨ Membranous part: Smallest part. Placed between the tricuspid leaflets (septal and anterior). The aortic cusps (right and non coronary) lie above this region.

Anatomical types of VSD (as seen from the RV)

- ⇨ Perimembranous: Also called conoventricular VSD or Infracristal VSD. MC type of VSD (80%). Lies below the aortic valve at the LVOT. Abnormal septal tricuspid leaflet seen (pouches/aneurysm). Further subclassified as inlet VSD, outlet VSD, muscular VSD. LV to RA defect may be associated (Gerbode defect).
- ⇨ Supracristal: Also called subarterial, doubly committed, outlet VSD, infundibular or subpulmonic VSD. Constitutes around 8% of the VSDs. Lies below the pulmonary valve. Commonly associated with AR due to aortic valve prolapse (right cusp > non coronary cusp). The presence of AR in VSD is an indication for early surgery. This type is common in Asian populations.
- ⇨ Muscular VSD: 2nd MC (5 - 20%). Can be central, marginal or apical depending on the location. "Swiss-cheese" defects are multiple muscular VSDs together.
- ⇨ Inlet VSD: Lies at the AV septum (endocardial cushion). Constitutes 5-12% of the VSDs. Lies below the TV and usually associated with AV valve abnormalities.

Pathophysiology of VSD

- ⇨ Shunting of blood (either L→R or R→L in Eisenmenger's syndrome) ⇨ PAH over prolonged period of time ⇨ Congestive cardiac failure.

It is the size of the VSD and the pulmonary vascular resistance that determines the state of the murmur and the clinical picture in VSD.

The associated lesions and the systemic vascular resistance are the other additional determinants.

One fact about VSD is that, when we think of VSD the primary thing in our mind is the L→R shunt. But, it is noteworthy that the LA and LV are the chambers that are affected and not the RV. This is because the shunting of blood from LV to RV occurs in systole when both the ventricles are contracting. Hence, the shunted blood is directly poured to the PA which is then returned to the LA via the PV. This leads to enlargement of the LA and LV that ultimately receives the extra amount of blood. This can lead to LV failure in early life.

Restrictive VSD

The VSD defect itself acts as the resisting force to limit the L→R shunt. RVSP<LVSP when there is no RVOT obstruction.

Non-restrictive VSD

The L→R shunting is not resisted which leads to equalization of the LV and RV systolic pressures and hence the PVR is the deciding factor for the amount of L→R shunt.

Other parameters used to classify VSDs

- ⇨ Diameter of the VSD relative to the diameter of the normal aortic annulus
- ⇨ RVSP/LVSP (determined at cardiac catheterization)
- ⇨ Pulmonary blood flow/Systemic blood flow (Qp/Qs) (determined at cardiac catheterization)

Small VSD

- ⇨ VSD diameter < 1/3rd the diameter of the normal aortic annulus
- ⇨ RVSP/LVSP < 0.3
- ⇨ Qp/Qs < 1.4

Moderate VSD

- ⇨ VSD diameter 1/3rd to 2/3rd the diameter of the normal aortic annulus
- ⇨ RVSP/LVSP > 0.3
- ⇨ Qp/Qs - 1.4-2.0

Large VSD

- ⇨ VSD diameter > 2/3rd the diameter of the normal aortic annulus
- ⇨ RVSP/LVSP > 0.3
- ⇨ Qp/Qs > 2.0

Eisenmenger's syndrome

⇨ RVSP/LVSP ≑ 1

⇨ Qp/Qs < 1.4

Murmur of VSD

Timing of the murmur:

⇨ The classical murmur of VSD is PSM (small or moderate VSD) which indicates a sustained pressure difference between the LV and RV.

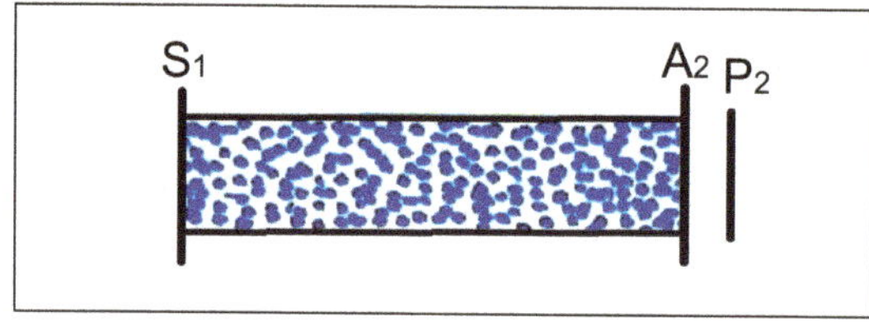

Fig. 15.9

⇨ However, as stated earlier it is the size of the VSD and the PVR that primarily determines the murmur. Hence, a restrictive VSD can produce a long and loud murmur, but a large non-restrictive VSD may not produce PSM.

VSD without PSM

Muscular VSD (closes at the later part of systole), large VSD(produces ESM), very minute VSD, raised RV pressure (PS, MR, PAH, etc).

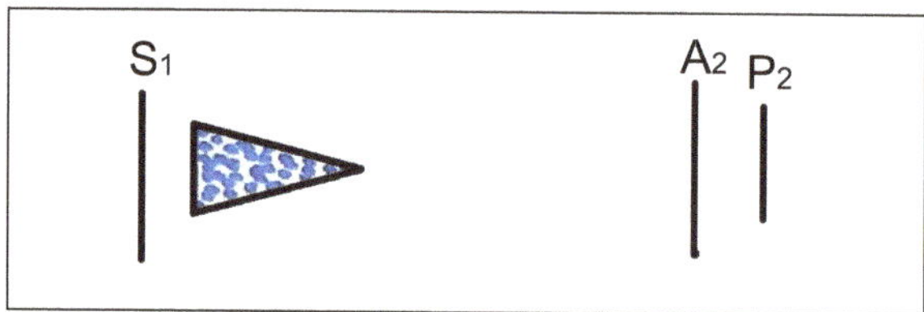

Fig. 15.10: Small muscular VSD.

Small muscular VSD

⇨ As pulmonary hypertension develops, the PSM changes to an ESM or completely disappears.

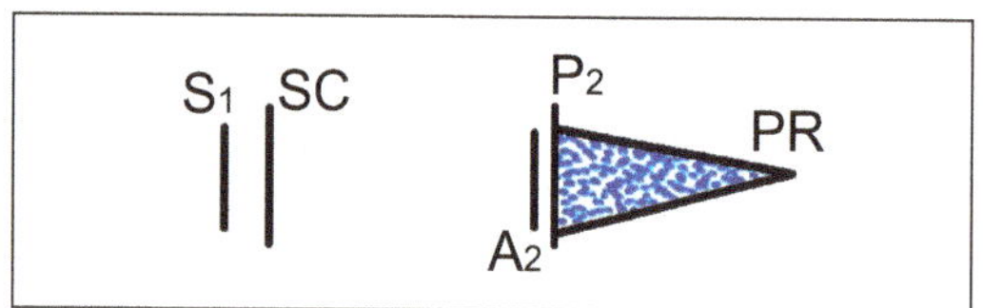

Fig. 15.11: VSD with Eisenmenger syndrome.

⇨ A coexisting PS can make the murmur disappear.

⇨ A coexisting small PDA or RSOV can mask the PSM of VSD by their continuous murmur (CM).

Area of best audibility and radiation

⇨ Left 2nd to 4th ICS without significant radiation.

⇨ Infundibular/supracristal VSD: Pulmonary area and radiating to the left infraclavicular region.

⇨ VSD with L-TGA: Apex

⇨ Gerbode's defect may radiate to the right side of the sternum.

Grade

⇨ > 4/6 with thrill.

Character

⇨ Rough

⇨ MR and TR murmurs are blowing in nature.

Dynamic auscultation

⇨ Murmur ↑ on expiration and ↓ on inspiration and with amyl nitrate.

JVP in VSD

⇨ Mean JVP ↑

⇨ Prominent a waves in VSD with associated PS

⇨ Prominent v waves with rapid y descent and absent x descent in associated TR or LV→RA type VSD (Gerbode's defect).

Arterial pulse In VSD

⇨ Restrictive defect: brisk arterial pulse

⇨ Large nonrestrictive VSD with CCF: weak arterial pulse

⇨ Eisenmenger's syndrome: Normal arterial pulse (since SV is normal).

Precordial palpation in VSD

⇨ Palpable thrill at left 3rd or 4th ICS.

⇨ Palpable P2

⇨ Parasternal heave due to RVH.

⇨ Apex is hyperdynamic, but may become sustained with the development of heart failure or when there is associated MR.

Acquired VSD

⇨ Commonly seen after anterior wall MI.

⇨ Leads to death in upto 5%.

⇨ Very common after the first MI.

⇨ ECG may show 3^0 AV block or RBBB.

⇨ A new onset VSD type murmur in a post MI patient above 40 years of age should raise the suspicion of a septal rupture.

Mimickers of VSD murmur

⇨ AS

⇨ TR

⇨ MR

⇨ PS

References

- Clinical examination in cardiology; 2nd edition; B N VIJAY RAGHAWA RAO.
- Ind J Car Dis Wom 2019;4:165-174;Maddury Jyotsna; Systolic Murmurs.
- Circulation,VolumeXVII, April1958;AUBREY LEATHAM, M.B; Systolic Murmurs.
- Synopsis of cardiac physical diagnosis; 2nd edition; Jonathan Abrams.
- Clinical methods in cardiology by B Soma Raju.
- Clinical Methods: The History, Physical, and Laboratory Examinations. 3rd edition. Chapter 26 Systolic Murmurs by MARTIN A. ALPERT.
- Nishimura et al. JACC Vol. 63, No. 22, 2014 AHA/ACC Valvular Heart Disease Guideline June 10, 2014:e57-185.
- The art and science of cardiac physical examination; 2nd edition; Narasimhan Ranganathan.
- J Pediatr (Rio J) 2003;79 Suppl 1:S87-S96: heart defects, congenital, heart auscultation, heart Murmurs; Assessment of heart murmurs in childhood by Maria Elisabeth B.A. Kobinger.
- Harrison's principles of Internal medicine, 18th edition, Page 1539, Mitral regurgitation.
- Ventricular Septal Defects by Dr. Vasco Rolo,Dr. Isabeau Walker,Dr. Kate Wilson; P A E D I A T R I C A N A E S T H E S I A Tutorial 316 ;1st JUNE 2015.
- Perloff's Clinical recognition of Congenital heart disease by Joseph K. Perloff and Ariane J. Marelli; 6th edition; Chapter 17 Ventricular septal defect.

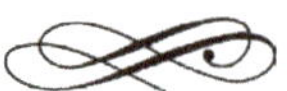

CHAPTER

16 Diastolic Murmurs

Murmur starts at or just after S2, but ending before the next S1.

Diastolic murmurs are further sub-classified as:-

- **Early diastolic (EDM):** Starts at or just after S2. Usually associated with fall of ventricular pressures below the great arteries (aorta or PA). Usually high pitched, with a blowing and decrescendo character reflecting pressure change. The murmur is loud due to a big regurgitant volume from the great arteries to the respective ventricles. Usually EDM occurs due to damage to the semilunar valves.
- **Mid diastolic (MDM):** Starts after S2 and stops before S1. Usually low pitched and associated with diseased AV valves (mitral and tricuspid) when there is a discrepency between AV valve area and the ventricular diastolic blood flow. However, sometimes even normal AV valves can have MDM when the diastolic blood flow is increased, eg; VSD, PDA, ASD.
- **Late diastolic (LDM)/Presystolic:** Occurs just before S1 during the rapid ventricular filling phase preceded by the atrial contraction. Usually associated with MS or TS but, sometimes also seen with atrial myxomas.

  LDM can also be seen in atrial fibrillation where there is a sustained diastolic pressure gradient that leads to persistent flow across the MV in diastole.

EARLY DIASTOLIC MURMUR (EDM)

Usually occurs in:

- Aortic regurgitation (AR)
- Pulmonary regurgitation (PR)

CHRONIC AORTIC REGURGITATION (AR)

The aortic valve apparatus includes:

- Valve cusps
- Valve annulus
- Commissures
- Sinus of Valsalva
- Proper LV functioning

Any breach in the normal functioning of the constituent aortic valve apparatus may lead to AR.

Etiology of AR

- ⇨ RHD (MC)
- ⇨ IE
- ⇨ Syphilis
- ⇨ Cystic medial necrosis
- ⇨ Bicuspid aortic valve
- ⇨ Aortic root diseases: Sinus of Valsalva aneurysm, ankylosing spondylitis, Marfan's syndrome, idiopathic dilatation, Ehlers-Danlos syndrome, aortitis.

Acute AR: Trauma, IE, aortic dissection.

The pathophysiology of AR

AR is a state of volume overload, where additional blood is regurgitated back to the LV either due to diseased aortic valve or dilatation of the proximal aorta.

Initially the LV overcomes this volume overload by increasing the compliance and rigorously ejecting this blood leading to ↑SV and a normal LV filling pressure.

With the passage of time, there is eccentric hypertrophy of the LV with dilatation but little chamber hypertrophy.

As the disease progresses and severe AR sets in the LV compliance decreases with increasing LV filling pressure and finally cardiac failure.

In acute onset AR, the LV is suddenly loaded with the diastolic overload and cannot adjust to this abrupt phenomenon. As a result there is severely raised LV filling pressure with fall in the CO and rapid congestive heart failure (poor prognosis). There is also systemic vasoconstriction which attenuates the peripheral signs of AR.

Murmur of AR

Classically EDM starting with the A2 component of S2 with a blowing, high pitched quality and decrescendo configuration. The murmur tapers in the diastole.

The murmur length depends on the amount of the regurgitation.

Even a faint murmur of AR is suggestive of a definite heart disease.

Sometimes may be confused with the EDM of PR which starts a little later with the P2 component.

Heard best with the diaphragm of the stethoscope (unlike DM of MS at the apex which is best heard with the bell of the stethoscope).

A systolic ejection murmur may occur in moderate to severe AR due to the increased SV that is ejected with great force. This murmur can be upto 3-4/6 grade. It may be sometimes confused with a murmur of associated AS. However, with a diastolic BP of < 40-50 mmHg, AS is easily ruled out.

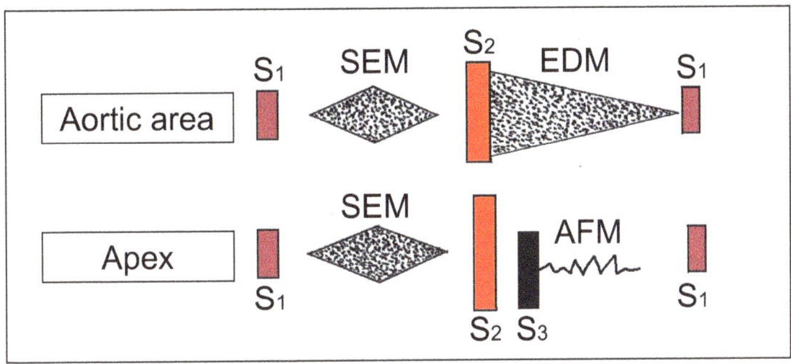

Fig. 16.1: Chronic AR.

Area of best audibility

⇨ Rheumatic AR: left sternal border (sometimes also at the aortic area and cardiac apex)

⇨ Syphilitic AR (aortic root involvement): sternal border on the right (sometimes also at the cardiac apex and left sternal border)

AR due to valvular involvement (RHD, IE, BAV) ⇨ murmur along the left sternal border.

AR due to root involvement, dissection of the aorta, aneurysm of the sinus of Valsalva, right cusp perforation⇨ murmur along the right sternal border.

Contour/character of the murmur

⇨ Since the pressure difference in the diastole is high between aorta and LV, the murmur has a high pitch with a blowing character, but is soft. The murmur is rarely > 4/6 grade.

⇨ Vegetations on the aortic valve due to IE: murmur has a musical quality.

⇨ Syphilitic AR with retroverted cusps: murmur has a rough quality and is associated with a thrill.

Length of the murmur

⇨ Length of the murmur indicates how long the pressure difference has been maintained between the aorta and the LV during diastole.

⇨ The length of the murmur is directly proportional to the amount of aortic valve damage and the aortic pressure.

⇨ It is inversely proportional to the LVEDP.

⇨ Short EDM: Mild AR

Long EDM: Severe AR

However, there are certain clinical scenarios where in spite of a severe AR, there is a very short murmur or at times no murmur at all. These conditions are:

⇨ LV dysfunction

⇨ AR of acute onset

⇨ ↑HR

⇨ ↓BP

⇨ Pregnancy

Dynamic auscultation

⇨ For AR murmur auscultation, the patient is positioned in a sitting and leaning forward posture with the breath held in full expiration.

⇨ Sustained handgrip, phenylephrine, squatting or Valsalva (strain phase) may unmask a faint murmur of AR by increasing the systemic resistance.

⇨ Amyl nitrate reduces the intensity of the murmur.

Arterial BP

⇨ With worsening AR, the SBP↑ and the DBP↓ and there is a wide pulse pressure.

⇨ The falling DBP is a better indicator for the severity of the AR. It may go down to even 40 mmHg in severe AR.

⇨ The SBP may rise to 150 mmHg, but usually do not cross above 160 mmHg until the patient is a known hypertensive.

Carotid pulse

⇨ High amplitude, bounding pulse due to increased SV with a quick collapsing nature due to rapid diastolic run-off into the LV and ↓ SVR.

⇨ Corrigan's sign: visible carotid pulsations.

⇨ Severe AR or AR with AS: Bisferiens pulse.

AR associated peripheral signs indicating wide pulse pressure

Peripheral signs indicate severe AR always, if there is no heart failure. Occurrence of heart failure would ↓ the CO which may then mask these peripheral findings.

(1) ↑ sweating with warm skin due to systemic vasodilation.

(2) Hill's sign: Popliteal SBP > Brachial SBP by at least 20-40 mmHg (mild AR), 40-60 mmHg (moderate AR), > 60 mmHg (severe AR).

(3) Bisferiens pulse.

(4) Corrigan's sign.

(5) Palmar flushing in systole.

(6) Traube's sign: On auscultation of the femoral arteries, a pistol shot-like sound is heard. (In severe TR, pistol shot-like sound can be heard over the femoral veins).

(7) Duroziez's sign: Systolic murmur on proximal compression of femoral artery (due to ↑ diastolic reversal of flow).

(8) Duroziez's murmur: Diastolic murmur on distal compression (with the stethoscope edge).

(9) Quincke's sign/pulsations: Sequential capillary pulsations on light pressure over the nail bed or the lips (with a glass slide).

(10) de Musset's sign: Head bobbing, synchronous with the cardiac beats as a result of ballistic effect due to severe regurgitation.

(11) Water hammer pulse (discussed earlier).

(12) Muller's sign: Uvular pulsations, synchronous with the cardiac systole.

(13) Landolfi's sign: Pupillary contraction in systole and dilation in diastole due to ↑ SV.

(14) Becker's sign: Pulsating retinal arteries.

(15) Rosenbach's sign: Pulsating liver.

(16) Gerhardt's sign: Splenomegaly with pulsations.

(17) Light house sign: The forehead shows alternating flushes and blanching.

Precordium in AR

⇨ Mild to moderate AR: Hyperdynamic precordium

⇨ Severe AR: Hyperdynamic precordium with displacement of the cardiac apex down and out.

⇨ Severe AR with LV dysfunction: Sustained apical impulse.

Cardiac sounds in AR

⇨ S1: Normal in mild AR; soft in severe AR. A loud S1 at the base in patients of AR is actually aortic ejection click rather than S1.

⇨ S2: May be soft due to poor leaflet vibrations; single S2 in severe AR. Loud A2 in AR due to syphilis.

⇨ S3: Common in severe AR; occurs due to ↑diastolic volume with dilatation and dysfunction of the LV. Its presence indicates a bad prognosis.

⇨ S4: Uncommon

⇨ Aortic ejection click: Valvular click in BAV; vascular click in dilated root associated AR.

Differences between AR and PR

	AR	PR
Area of best audibility	Right 2nd ICS	Left 2nd ICS
Best posture	Sitting and leaning forward	Supine
Wide pulse pressure	Seen	Not seen
Cardiac apex	Hyperdynamic	RV heave
Relation to respiration	Nil	Louder with inspiration
Peripheral signs	Present	Absent
S2	May be soft	Loud P2
Ventricular size	LVH	RVH

Austin-Flint murmur (AFM)

It is a low pitched, apical murmur occurring in early to mid diastole with a presystolic component that extends or ends just at S1. It mimics the MDM of MS to a great extent. It is heard with the bell of the stethoscope.

Many times, the AFM merges with S3 and produces a loud mid diastolic sound/murmur.

AFM is an indicator that a large amount of blood is regurgitating back to the LV and the AR fraction is > 50% with a raised LVEDV.

Usually the peripheral signs of severe grade AR are present along with FM.

It occurs due to the large aortic regurgitant volume hitting the AML and preventing its proper opening during diastole.

However, the murmur occurs only when the MV is about to close.

Sustained handgrip ↑ the murmur while amyl nitrate ↓ it.

In severe AR, when MV closes prematurely in the later part of diastole, the presystolic component is absent.

Points of differentiation between AFM and MS

	AFM	MS
Opening snap	No	Yes
Loud S1	No	Yes
Thrill	Less common	Common
Amyl nitrate	Murmur↓	Murmur↑

(Continued)

Sustained handgrip	Murmur↑	No specific response
Vasopressor drugs	Murmur↑	No specific response
Atrial fibrillation	Absent	Common
S3	Present	Absent always
LV hypertrophy	Seen	Absent
RV hypertrophy	Absent	Seen
PAH	Unusual	Common

ACUTE AR

Causes and clinical correlation

- IE (fever)
- Perforation (h/o trauma)
- Dissection (acute onset chest and back pain)
- Myxomatous degeneration
- PTCA (presenting as sudden drop of diastolic BP initially with increased PA pressures).

Pathophysiology

Sudden regurgitation of blood from aorta to the LV ⇨ the normal LV fails to adjust ⇨ ↑LV filling pressure and LVF ⇨ soft S1 due to MV closing prematurely and there is cold clammy limbs due to systemic vasoconstriction and sinus tachycardia with shortening of diastole.

The murmur of acute AR is short due to raised LV filling pressure and is usually grade 3/6 or less.

Blood pressure in acute AR

- SBP doesn't increases
- DBP may or may not decrease
- Normal pulse pressure

Pulse in acute AR

- No pulsus bisferiens
- No peripheral signs

JVP in acute AR

- Usually raised with associated TR due to RVF.

Precordium in acute AR

⇨ Usually normal, but RV heave may be present if there is LVF leading to ↑PASP.

Cardiac sounds in acute AR

⇨ S1 soft; P2 may be normal or loud; S3 commonly present.

Murmurs of acute AR

⇨ Diastolic murmur is short and soft

⇨ Austin-Flintt murmur is mid-diastolic always without presystolic component.

⇨ Systolic murmur usually present, although it may be soft.

⇨ MR murmur usually present.

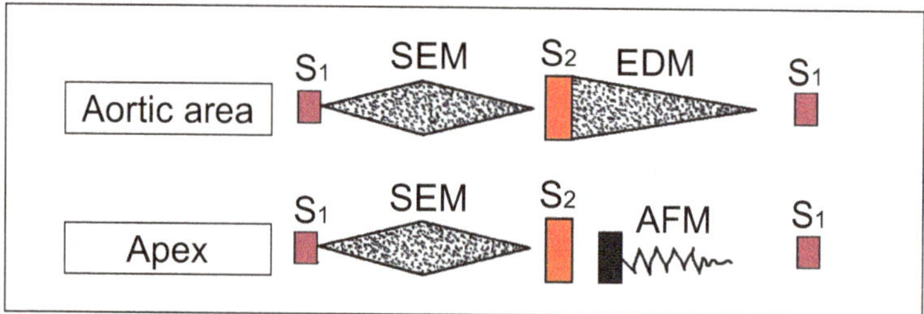

Fig. 16.2: Acute AR.

PULMONARY REGURGITATION (PR)

While discussing PR, it is essential to describe whether the PR is associated with pulmonary hypertension (**Graham Steell murmur**) or there is no pulmonary hypertension (normal pulmonary artery pressure).

Causes of normal pressure PR (without PAH)

⇨ Congenital

⇨ Idiopathic PA dilatation

⇨ Pulmonary valve dysplasia with PS

⇨ Absent pulmonary valves in TOF

⇨ Carcinoid syndrome

⇨ IE

⇨ RHD

⇨ Post surgical trauma

⇨ Post surgical repair of TOF

Some distinctions and descriptions of PR with PAH and PR with normal PAP

	PR with PAH	PR with normal PAP
Timing	Early diastolic murmur (EDM)	MID diastolic murmur (MDM)
Pitch and contour	High frequency, decrescendo murmur; sometimes rough (where it may be confused with the systolic murmur of VSD or PS).	Low frequency, rumbling. With absent pulmonary valves (TOF), there may be an associated ejection systolic murmur due to narrowing of annulus.
Length of the murmur	Long; sometimes pandiastolic if the PADP > 50mmHg.	Short usually (PADP ≑ 10-14 mmHg).
Area of best audibility	Pulmonary area; sometimes at the cardiac apex there is RV enlargement.	Pulmonary area only; rarely at the left border of the sternum.
Associated diastolic thrill	Sometimes present	Absent
On Inspiration	Murmur may ↑	Murmur ↑ (However, the murmur of TS ↑even further on inspiration).
Standing posture	Murmur ↓ but remains the same in presence of RVF.	Murmur ↓
Supine posture	Murmur ↑	Murmur ↑
Sustained handgrip	No change	No change
Vasopressor	No change	No change
RV S3 and S4	Yes	No
Pulmonary hypertension	Yes	No
Associated IE	No	Yes
Loud P2	Yes	No (Soft P2)
TR	Common	No
Right Austin Flint murmur	Yes	No
Pulmonary vascular ejection click	Yes	No
RVH	Yes	No
JVP showing prominent a wave	Yes	No

GRAHAM STEELL MURMUR (GSM)

GSM of PR always indicates a raised pulmonary artery pressure above the systemic range.

GSM occurring in valvular heart disease, as a rule indicates severe grade MS.

When patients of L→R shunts develop GSM, it indicates that the defect is not operable.

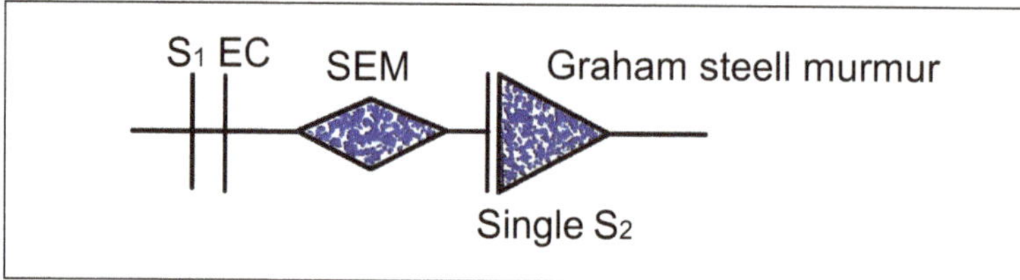

Fig. 16.3

However, GSM may occur without PAH in ASD patients, but there is associated dilatation of the pulmonary artery which can give rise to the EDM due to ↑ pulmonary blood flow.

In Eisenmenger's syndrome, there is GSM along with cyanosis.

Cyanotic heart diseases with pulmonary hypertension like TGA, TAPVC, DORV may sometimes develop GSM.

MID DIASTOLIC MURMUR (MDM)

MDM occur in conditions like:

⇨ Mitral stenosis

⇨ Tricuspid stenosis

⇨ Myxomas (left and right)

⇨ Carey Coomb's murmur

⇨ Murmur due to ↑ flow such as in ASD, VSD, MR, TR, PDA, etc.

⇨ Carcinoid syndrome

⇨ Austin Flint murmur (described earlier)

MITRAL STENOSIS (MS)

RHD is the MC cause of MS, occurring in nearly 40% of the patients.

The damage to the MV apparatus usually starts at the commissures with fusion and narrowing of the orifice which gives the typical "fish mouth appearance".

There is thickening of the valve leaflets with calcification later.

MS and onset of symptoms

⇨ Normal Mitral valve area (MVA) - 4 to 6 cm^2

⇨ MVA<50% of the normal (2 to 2.5 cm^2) - symptoms starts

⇨ MVA 1.5 to 2.0 cm^2 - fatigue and breathlessness occurs

⇨ MVA < 1.5 cm^2 - hemodynamic consequences start like paroxysmal nocturnal dyspnea.

⇨ MVA < 1.0 cm^2 - LA has to pump the blood at a pressure > 25 mmHg to maintain normal circulation. Patients can develop orthopnea.

Echocardiographic grading of the severity of MS

Depending on the mean gradient across the MV:

⇨ Mild: < 5 mmHg

⇨ Moderate: 5-10 mmHg

⇨ Severe: > 10 mmHg

Depending on the MVA:

⇨ Mild to moderate (progressive MS): >1.5 cm^2

⇨ Severe: ≤ 1.5 cm^2

⇨ Very severe: ≤ 1 cm^2

Mitral stenosis murmur

Timing of the murmur

⇨ Mid diastolic with presystolic accentuation (murmur) (Pre-SM).

⇨ The murmur starts after S2 and ends before S1.

⇨ The murmur can occasionally be early diastolic in conditions of MS with PAH with disease of the aortic valve where the P2 is delayed and the A2 is ↓.

⇨ The presystolic accentuation occurs due to (1) a sustained gradient between the LA and LV, (2) contraction of the LA and (3) ↓in MVA due to presystolic contraction of the LV.

⇨ Sometimes the atrial gallop in HCM is so loud that it may be confused as presystolic accentuation. Similarly, severe PS can cause a right sided atrial gallop which may be wrongly interpreted as presystolic accentuation.

Absent presystolic accentuation

- Very mild MS
- Atrial fibrillation (AF)
- Long PR interval
- Dysfunction of the LV or raised LVEDP
- ↓HR

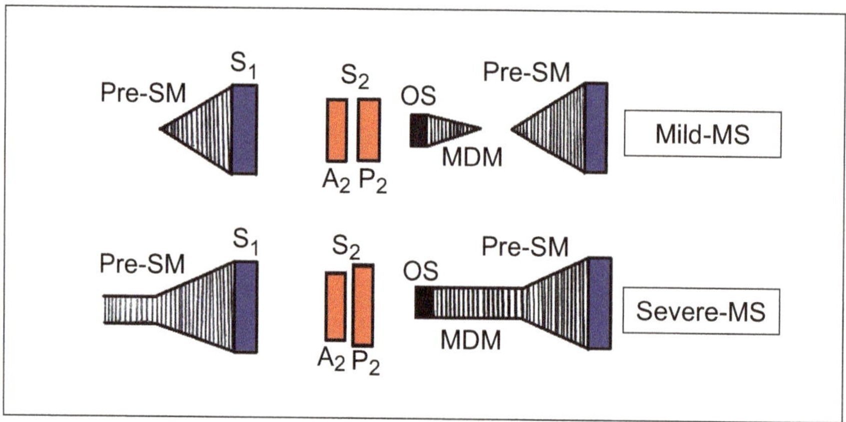

Fig. 16.4

Area of best audibility

⇨ Best heard at the cardiac apex without significant radiation to other areas (due to lower pitch).

⇨ Usually heard in the left lateral decubitus posture with the bell of the stethoscope in held expiration.

⇨ Rarely, the murmur may be best heard at sites other than the apex like TA, PA, left border of the sternum (due to short AML and abnormal jet direction), xiphisternum (in COPD patients).

Pitch, contour and length

⇨ The murmur is rough with a rumbling quality and the pitch is low due to a lower pressure gradient between the LA and LV (maximum upto 30 mmHg in LA in severe MS).

⇨ There is early diastolic decrescendo and late diastolic crescendo nature of the murmur.

⇨ A loud murmur with thrill is suggestive of non-calcified and pliable valve leaflets that create vibrations of lower frequencies.

⇨ The murmur length is directly proportional to the severity of the stenosis, when the CO, HR, LA pressure, cardiac rhythm and the LV filling pressures are within the normal range.

⇨ Hence, when the above mentioned parameters are deranged, the length of the murmur doesn't correlate with the disease severity. These conditions are:

- Altered heart rate → Tachycardia (↑length), bradycardia (↓length)
- Altered CO → RV dysfunction (↓CO, ↓length), PAH (↓CO, ↓length), hyperdynamic states (↑CO, ↑length).
- Raised LV filling pressure → IHD, HTN, aortic disease, etc. (↓length)
- Cardiac arrhythmia → Atrial fibrillation (length variable).

Loud S1 in MS

⇨ S1 is loud because there is a presystolic gradient between the LA and LV which keeps the valve leaflets wide apart just prior to the onset of systole.

⇨ With the onset of systole, there is an ↑ dp/dt which closes the widely separated valve leaflets with great velocity causing the ↑ S1.

⇨ However, for S1 to be loud in MS, the valves should be mobile and thick, else a severely calcified MS may lead to an absent S1 also.

⇨ Loud S1 is the most distinct feature of MS which helps to confirm the diagnosis.

⇨ If the patient presents with all findings of MS, but there is no loud S1, we should consider other possible diagnoses like:

- AFM (Mid diastolic murmur at the cardiac apex in severe AR)
- Severely calcified MV leaflets
- LA myxoma
- Severe MR or severe AR in association with MS
- Very severe MR alone (Mid diastolic murmur)

Opening snap (OS)

High frequency, early diastolic, clicking sound caused by the sudden stoppage of the opening AV valves, especially when the valve leaflets are thick and deformed but mobile and is associated with an ↑ LAP or ↑ flow across the valves.

Characteristics of Opening snap

Frequency: High

Occurs in early diastole following A2 after an average interval of about 60-120 ms.

Auscultation: With the diaphragm of the stethoscope just inside of the apex beat for Mitral OS and lower left sternum for Tricuspid OS. The mitral OS is better heard after exercise and it does not change with respiration. The OS is usually followed by the MDM which becomes prominent with exercise.

> **NOTE**
>
> The mitral OS may sometimes be heard at the pulmonary area and may be confused with a split S2.

Etiopathogenesis of OS

(1) AV valve stenosis ⇨ MS, TS

(2) ↑flow across the AV valves with great force ⇨

Mitral valve: MR, large VSD, HOCM, MVP, hyperthyroidism, PDA.

Tricuspid valve: Large ASD, TR, Ebstein anomaly.

Conditions where OS can be missed even in the presence of a significant MS

⇨ Very severely calcified, immobile mitral valves

⇨ Severe MR

⇨ Severe AR

⇨ Severe AS

⇨ LV dysfunction or LVF with CAD

⇨ When OS is heard at the pulmonary area, where it is misinterpreted as a split S2.

The A2-OS interval

Now, thinking of the sequences of the cardiac cycle, we know:-

With the end of systole→beginning of isovolumetric relaxation (diastole)→closure of the aortic valve (A2) →LA-LV pressure crossover (where LA pressure exceeds LV pressure)→opening of the mitral valve (to produce OS).

From the above sequence, it is clear that it is the LAP that can influence the MV opening time. If the LAP is raised, the LA-LV pressure crossover time is reduced and the MV opens immediately following the A2, i.e.; the A2-OS time decreases.

Since the LAP increases with the increasing severity of MS, the A2-OS interval has an inverse relation to the MS severity.........more the severity of MS, lesser is the A2-OS interval and vice versa.

Although the A2-OS interval also depends on the aortic pressure level, and the rate of isovolumetric relaxation, the LAP is the most important factor that influences the A2-OS interval.

The normal A2-OS interval ranges between 50-120 ms.

In mild MS: A2-OS interval is > 120 ms with a rough LAP of around 14-15 mmHg.

In moderate MS: A2-OS interval is around 80-100 ms with a rough LAP of around 20-22 mmHg.

In severe MS: A2-OS interval is around 50-70 ms with a rough LAP of around 24-25 mmHg.

However, there are numerous factors that can affect the A2-OS interval. Some of them are enumerated below:-

(1) Heart rate (HR):

↑HR ⇨ ↓A2-OS interval because of the shortened diastole.

↓HR ⇨ ↑A2-OS interval because of the prolonged diastole.

(2) Time of aortic closure (occurrence of A2):

Hypertension ⇨ ↑A2-OS interval because of early A2.

AS ⇨ ↓A2-OS interval because of delayed A2.

AR ⇨ ↑A2-OS interval because of early A2.

(3) Low LAP:

↑A2-OS interval as seen in RV dysfunction, TR, PAH, etc.

(4) ↑LA-LV pressure crossover time (↑LVEDP):

↑A2-OS interval in conditions like IHD, LV dysfunction in cardiomyopathies, etc.

Differences between A2-OS and A2-P2

	A2-OS	A2-P2
Best heard at	Just inside the apex	Pulmonary area
Time interval	50-120 ms	< 30 ms
Posture effect	Widens on standing	Narrows on standing
Respiratory variation	No change for mitral OS.	Widens on inspiration

> **NOTE**
>
> We must remember that in MS there is a reverse relationship between the length of the murmur and the A2-OS interval. This means that in severe MS, the length of the murmur increases and the A2-OS interval shortens and vice versa.
>
> A concordant relationship is seen usually in LA myxoma.

JVP in MS

⇨ Usually normal

⇨ With the development of PAH there is prominent a wave, and with the presence of TR there is prominent cv wave.

Precordium in MS

⇨ Diastolic thrill - apex

⇨ LV: underfilled and does not produce any abnormality.

⇨ Parasternal heave present. In severe cases, RV forms the apex.

⇨ Palpable P2 at the pulmonary area (PA).

Dynamic auscultation

Respiration:- The murmur ↑ in expiration due to ↑ venous return (VR) to the left side of the heart.

False positive Carvallo's sign is an ↑ in the murmur during inspiration, which may occur as a result of a shortened diastole secondary to inspiration induced ↑ in the HR.

Exercise:- ↑ the murmur due to ↑ CO.

Posture:- The murmur ↓ on standing as a result of ↓ VR.

Amyl nitrate:- ↑ the murmur due ↑ HR.

Valsalva:- The murmur ↓.

Other causes of apical diastolic murmur

⇨ AFM

⇨ Very severe MR alone

⇨ Cor triatriatum

⇨ LA myxoma

⇨ Carey Coombs murmur

⇨ ASD

⇨ PDA

⇨ Hyperdynamic states.

TRICUSPID STENOSIS (TS)

RHD - MC cause.

TS is mostly associated with co-existing MS.

Females affected > males.

Etiology of TS

⇨ RHD

⇨ IE

⇨ Carcinoid syndrome

⇨ SLE

⇨ Ebstein's anomaly

⇨ Fabry's disease

⇨ Tumors (renal carcinoma, ovarian carcinoma)

⇨ RA myxoma

Pathophysiology of TS

⇨ In TS, there is a pressure gradient in diastole between RA→RV.

⇨ The RA pressure increases even with a mean gradient of 5 mmHg leading to congestive symptoms like ascites, peripheral edema and raised JVP.

JVP in TS

⇨ Prominent a wave; slow y descent.

The murmur of TS

Timing of the murmur

⇨ Presystolic murmur - MC component in TS

⇨ MDM may be present or absent (atrial fibrillation, associated MS, ongoing diuretic therapy, Ebstein's anomaly). However, the MDM of TS occurs slightly early in diastole which can be confused with the EDM of AR or PR. But the EDM of AR or PR doesn't ↑ with inspiration.

⇨ The MDM is similar to MS, but ↑ with deep inspiration which is the distinguishing feature.

⇨ Length of the murmur is directly proportional to the severity of stenosis except in Ebstein's anomaly and RHD with PAH.

Area of best audibility

⇨ Tricuspid area

⇨ RHD induced TS may be associated with RA enlargement in which case the murmur is best heard at the apex.

Contour

⇨ Rough, low frequency murmur with a rumbling quality.

⇨ This rough quality makes the murmur of TS often to be confused with pericardial rub.

Dynamic auscultation

⇨ Inspiration: murmur intensity ↑ (Carvallo's sign)

⇨ Leg raising with supine posture: murmur intensity ↑

⇨ Rapid breathing for 6-8 times: murmur intensity ↑ (due to accumulation of the ↑ VR).

Other causes of diastolic murmur occurring at the tricuspid valve level

⇨ ASD, PAPVC, Gerbode's defect, coronary artery fistula to RA (due to ↑flow)

⇨ Very severe TR

⇨ Mimicking murmurs at TA: AFM, MS, AR, pericardial rub.

Differences between murmurs of TS and MS

	MS	TS
Area of best audibility	Mitral area (Apex)	Tricuspid area
Duration of the murmur	Slightly lengthy	Shorter
Timing of the murmur	MDM with decrescendo - crescendo nature	Although MDM, but occurs slightly earlier in diastole
Contour	Rumbling	Scratch-like
Dynamic auscultation	↑ with exercise	↑ with inspiration

LEFT ATRIAL MYXOMA

⇨ Produces MDM mimicking MS.

⇨ The murmur is presystolic with crescendo nature.

⇨ The classical feature of LA myxoma murmur is the change in character and loudness with changing posture.

⇨ The murmur occurs once the myxoma sits on the mitral valve during the flow of blood from the LA to LV and the LV is about to contract.

CAREY COOMBS MURMUR

⇨ Seen in acute rheumatic fever.

⇨ The murmur occurs as ↑blood flow occurs across the edematous mitral valves (mitral valvulitis).

⇨ There is no OS.

⇨ Heard with bell of stethoscope in left lateral decubitus posture in expiration.

⇨ One more school of thoughts about the genesis of the murmur is that 1^0 AV blocks which are very common in rheumatic carditis causes a premature atrial contraction which sums up with the rapid ventricular filling phase and leads to the murmur.

PROSTHETIC VALVES

⇨ Bioprosthetic mitral valve may produce a DM in left lateral decubitus posture.

⇨ Bioprosthetic valves with degeneration or mechanical valves with thrombosis can cause MDM.

⇨ DM in caged ball prosthesis - abnormal.

DIASTOLIC MURMUR OF MR

⇨ Occurs in severe rheumatic MR, where a large amount of blood flows from the LA to LV leading to a functional MS.

⇨ The murmur is similar to that seen in MS, but the presystolic component is absent and there is presence of S3.

⇨ S1 is usually soft or absent.

Other causes of diastolic flow murmur at the MV level are:

- VSD
- PDA
- AV fistula
- Truncus arteriosus
- DORV
- Atresia of TV with associated PS
- Hyperdynamic states
- Very severe MR

DIASTOLIC MURMUR OF ASD

⇨ These are diastolic flow murmurs at the TV level due to L→ R shunt.

⇨ Medium to low frequency, best audible at the left lower sternum or at the apex if RV is enlarged.

⇨ S3 is usually present and there is absence of OS or presystolic accentuation.

⇨ No change occurs with inspiration.

⇨ This MDM is very specific (but not diagnostic) of ASD.

Other causes of MDM at the TV level are:

- RSOV
- PAPVC
- TAPVC
- Gerbode's defect
- Very severe TR
- AFM of right heart origin (severe PR)
- Atresia of MV

LATE DIASTOLIC MURMUR (LDM)/PRESYSTOLIC MURMUR

⇨ Presystolic murmur of MS

⇨ Presystolic murmur of TS

⇨ Short murmur in complete heart block called Rytand's murmur.

Other Diastolic murmurs

(1) Dock's murmur:

⇨ Seen in stenotic lesions of the left anterior descending (LAD) artery.

⇨ EDM.

⇨ Decrescendo in nature.

(2) Cole Cecil murmur:

⇨ When the EDM in AR is best audible at the axillary area.

(3) Cabot Locke Murmur:

⇨ Seen in hyperdynamic states like anemia where there is ↑ flow of blood through the left main coronary artery (LMCA) or LAD.

⇨ EDM.

⇨ Decrescendo in nature.

(4) Key Hodgkin's murmur:

⇨ Seen in syphilis with retroverted aortic leaflets.

⇨ EDM.

⇨ Decrescendo in nature.

References

- Manual of Practical Medicine By R Alagappan, 4th Edition.
- Clinical examination in cardiology; 2nd edition; B N Vijay Raghawa Rao.
- Synopsis of cardiac physical diagnosis; 2nd edition; Jonathan Abrams.
- Clinical methods in cardiology by B Soma Raju.
- Ind J Car Dis Wom 2019;4:228-232 ,The Diastolic Murmurs BY Amar Narayan Patnaik.
- The Echo Manual, 14th edition by Jae K. Oh, Chapter 13, Native valvular heart disease.
- Golamari R, Bhattacharya PT. Tricuspid Stenosis. [Updated 2020 Feb 4]. In: StatPearls [Internet]. Treasure Island (FL): StatPearls Publishing; 2020 Jan.
- Oxford medicine online;Chapter: Tricuspid stenosis Author(s): Michele De Bonis, and Patrizio Lancellotti;DOI: 10.1093/med/9780198784906.003.0770.

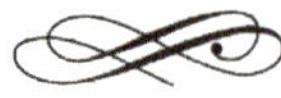

CHAPTER

17 Continuous Murmurs (CM)

A murmur that occupies the whole of systole and diastole with a constant character.

Care must be taken not to misinterpret a combination of systolic and diastolic murmur (mixed stenotic and regurgitant lesion) as a CM.

CM are caused by a constant blood flow during both systole and diastole from a high pressure/resistance chamber to a low pressure/resistance chamber.

Causes of CM

(1) Due to rapid flow of blood

- ⇨ Venous hum
- ⇨ Hyperthyroidism
- ⇨ Renal cell carcinoma
- ⇨ Mammary souffle
- ⇨ Alcoholic hepatitis
- ⇨ Hemangiomas

(2) Shunting from a high pressure to low pressure chamber

- ⇨ Aorta to PA shunting: PDA, truncus arteriosus, aortopulmonary window, pulmonary atresia, bronchiectasis, etc.
- ⇨ Aorta to the right side of the heart shunting: RSOV, coronary fistula.
- ⇨ L→R shunting in atria: MS with ASD (Lutembacher syndrome), atresia of MV with ASD.
- ⇨ AV fistula
- ⇨ Venovenous shunting: Portosystemic shunting, pulmonary vein anomaly.
- ⇨ Iatrogenic: After needle injury, post cardiac catheterization, post surgery etc.

(3) Severe arterial stenosis

- ⇨ COA
- ⇨ Peripheral (branch) pulmonary stenosis
- ⇨ Stenosis of Carotid artery
- ⇨ Stenosis of renal artery

⇨ Stenosis of femoral artery

⇨ Stenosis of coronary artery

⇨ Stenosis of mesenteric artery

PATENT DUCTUS ARTERIOSUS (PDA)

⇨ Incidence: 1:2000 to 1:5000 live births.

⇨ Ductus has two orifices/openings:

- pulmonary opening to the left of the pulmonary trunk bifurcation near the left branch origin
- aortic opening distal to the left subclavian artery origin.

⇨ The closure of the ductus commences from the pulmonary end.

⇨ Ductus arteriosus - 6th aortic arch

⇨ **Functional closure** (due to oxygen tension) begins 10-15 hours post birth as a result of the medial smooth muscle contraction and completes by the 2nd week of life.

⇨ **Anatomical closure** completes by the 2nd to 3rd week post birth due to medial necrosis and hemorrhage, leading to the formation of ligamentum arteriosum.

⇨ Spontaneous closure does not occur after 3 months of patency in a full term infant and after 1 year in a premature infant.

⇨ Large L→R shunt is considered significant hemodynamically.

⇨ R→L shunt is suggestive of severely raised pulmonary arterial pressure and is a contraindication to shunt closure as it may aggravate the RV failure.

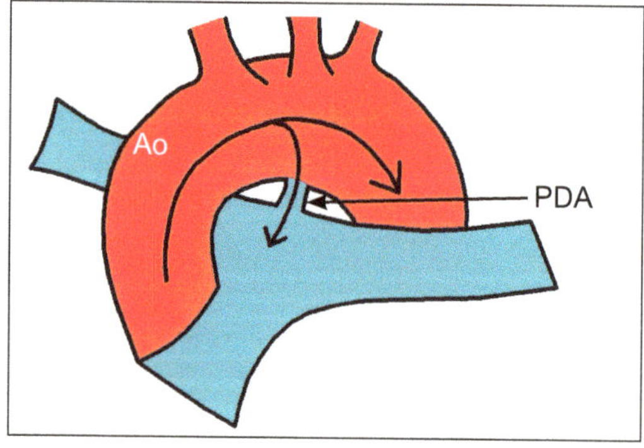

Fig. 17.1

The consequences of PDA depends on:

- size
- resistance in pulmonary vasculature

- acclimatization to the volume overload by the LV
- premature baby
- respiratory distress.

Risk factors for PDA:

⇨ Prematurity

⇨ Fluid overload

⇨ ARDS

⇨ Diuretics

⇨ Prolonged membrane rupture

⇨ Infections

⇨ Aminoglycoside antibiotics

Protective factors against PDA:

⇨ Corticosteroids given 24 hours prior to delivery

⇨ Hypertension in the mother

The murmur of PDA (Gibson's murmur)

Timing of the murmur

⇨ Continuous murmur with systolic peak (due to ↑ in descending aortic pressure later in systole) and diastolic tapering.

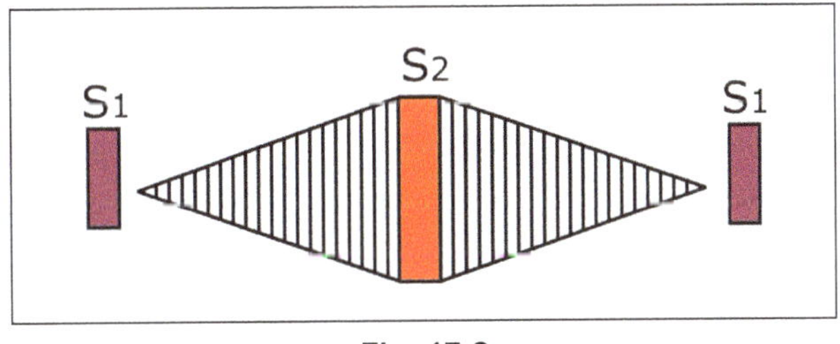

Fig. 17.2

⇨ The diastolic part is shorter always and as the pulmonary pressure ↑, it decreases further and finally vanishes followed by absence of the systolic component also. Hence, there may be no murmur in PDA once the pulmonary pressure equalizes the systemic pressure.

⇨ PDA with no continuous murmur occurs in conditions like:

- Severe PH
- A very large size ductus or a very small defect behaving like a valve

- Preductal COA
- Severe AS
- Large VSD
- MR with PAH
- MS with PAH

⇨ The murmur of PDA may at times be confused with murmur of VSD, but the clinical finding of a collapsing high volume pulse points towards PDA and not VSD.

Area of best audibility

⇨ Left 2nd ICS or Pulmonary area.

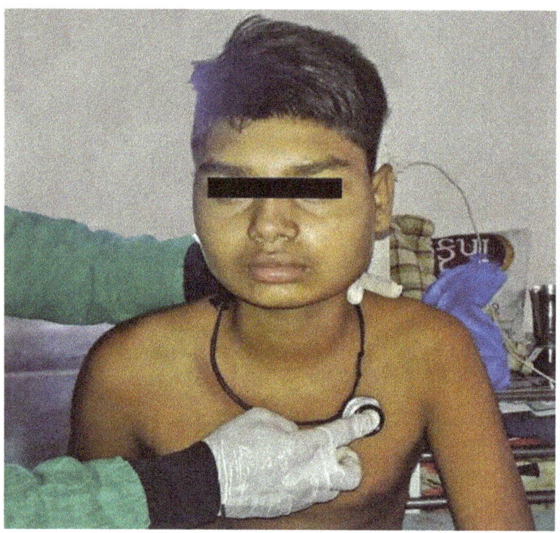

Fig. 17.3

⇨ The systolic part can be heard at the left lower border of the sternum, apex, right 2nd ICS or suprasternal area.

⇨ Diastolic part - pulmonary area.

⇨ Thrill - suprasternal area (differentiates from VSD)

Contour

⇨ Machinery in nature and associated with a thrill.

⇨ The diastolic and the systolic components have the same quality.

Dynamic auscultation

⇨ Expiration: murmur ↑

⇨ Sustained hand grip: murmur intensity and the duration ↑

⇨ Vasopressor drugs: murmur intensity and the duration ↑

⇨ Valsalva: Variable response.

Associated conditions to look for

⇨ Collapsing pulse: Supports a diagnosis of PDA.

⇨ Central cyanosis: Not seen with pure PDA alone. Search for other causes like bronchopulmonary collaterals.

⇨ Enlarged ventricles in PDA:

- LVH - common
- RVH - only if PAH is present (else think of RSOV).

⇨ Apical MDM in PDA: Indicates that the PAH is high flow related and can be operated.

RUPTURED SINUS OF VALSALVA ANEURYSM (RSOV)

⇨ Also called coronary sinus fistula.

⇨ Rare abnormality.

⇨ There is thinning of the walls of the aortic sinuses which forms an aneurysm resembling "wind sock" and which may rupture in the nearby chambers.

⇨ Congenital cause include a weak attachment between the aortic annulus and the aortic media.

⇨ Acquired causes include trauma, syphilis, IE, Behcet's disease, Marfan's syndrome.

⇨ Common associated cardiac lesions found in RSOV are VSD and AR.

⇨ Common in males and Asian population.

⇨ Symptoms include dyspnea, chest pain, and weakness.

⇨ Right sinus aneurysms are MC and mostly rupture into the RV or RA and rarely into the left chambers.

The murmur of RSOV

Timing of the murmur

⇨ CM - if the aneurysm ruptures into the atria as the pressure difference is great. The murmur - louder in diastole (differentiates from PDA). There is an associated thrill which is very much prominent.

⇨ Rupture into the RV may change the murmur as there may be a rise in the RVSP due to associated PAH.

⇨ The murmur is usually of the Grade 4/6.

Area of best audibility

⇨ Left 3rd or 4th ICS near to the sternal border with the patient sitting and leaning forward.

⇨ The murmur is heard at an area slightly lower than the area of audibility of PDA murmur.

Contour and length

⇨ The murmur is usually long with a superficial and rough character.

Radiation of the murmur

⇨ No conduction usually, but the diastolic part can be heard at the right side of the sternum as the diastolic runoff of aorta empties in the right sided chambers.

Dynamic auscultation

⇨ The murmur intensity does not change much with either respiration or vasopressors or sustained hand grip as there is a sustained pressure difference which is maintained throughout the cardiac cycle.

Heart sounds

⇨ S1 - normal

⇨ S2 - split with a loud P2.

Arterial pulse

⇨ Collapsing pulse with a wide pulse pressure.

JVP

⇨ Raised (due to right heart involvement)

Cardiac apex

⇨ Diffuse, hyperdynamic.

> **NOTE**
>
> Different scenarios of RSOV rupture:
>
> ⇨ RSOV rupturing into the RA, RV or LA will always produce a CM.
>
> ⇨ RSOV rupturing into the LV would produce an EDM.
>
> ⇨ PAH would abolish the systolic component of the murmur.
>
> ⇨ A coexisting VSD may superimpose and abolish the systolic component of the murmur, which may then sound as a to-and-fro murmur.
>
> ⇨ **"Tetrad of RSOV":** CM + Raised JVP + Collapsing pulse + Sudden chest pain.

VENOUS HUM

- The normal blood flow through the veins is noiseless.
- **Venous hum** is a type of CM which occurs when blood flows through the veins with increased velocity (hyperdynamic states) or when the viscosity of the blood reduces (anemia).
- **Physiologically,** venous hum can occur in children and pregnant females.
- It is heard with the bell of stethoscope between the heads of the sternocleidomastoid muscle with the patient sitting and the head turned to the other side.

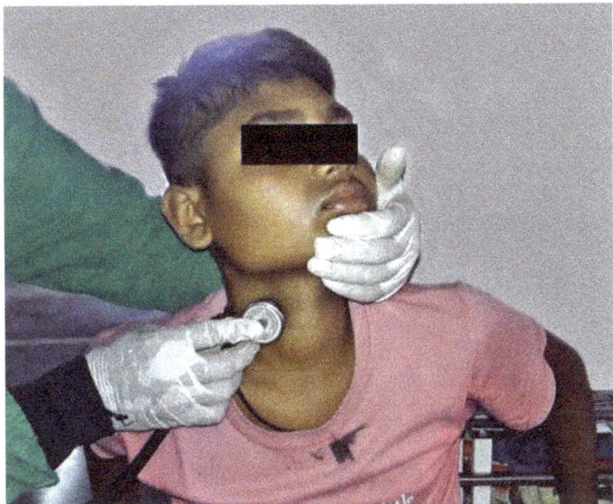

Fig. 17.4

- The murmur has a rough contour and sounds loud in diastole.
- The murmur disappears if the jugular vein is digitally compressed.

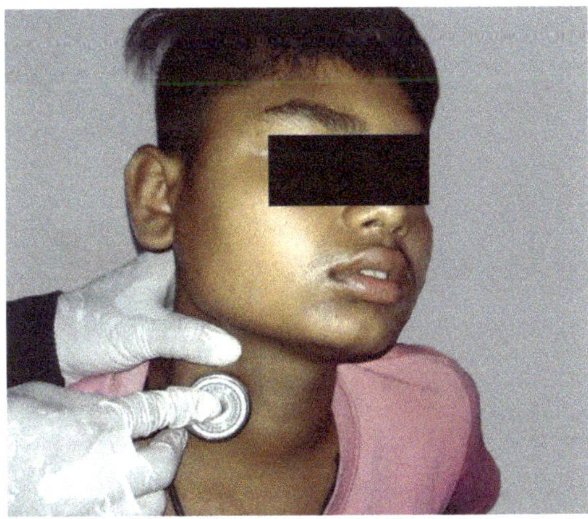

Fig. 17.5

⇨ **Adult with CCF and venous hum:** think of anemia or thyrotoxicosis.

⇨ **Child or infant with CCF and venous hum:** look for cranial bruit to r/o intracranial arteriovenous fistula.

MAMMARY SOUFFLE

⇨ A type of innocent CM with a loud systolic component.

⇨ Heard during the later months of pregnancy and lactating females.

⇨ The origin is arterial due to ↑ flow of blood to the breast tissues.

⇨ Best audible over the breasts from the 2nd to the 6th ICS, on both sides.

⇨ < 3/6 grade.

⇨ A distal strong pressure with stethoscope obliterates the murmur and distinguishes it from the murmur of PDA.

⇨ Light pressure ↑ the murmur.

⇨ Respiration and Valsalva has no influence on the murmur.

CORONARY CAMERAL FISTULA

⇨ Due to abnormalities occurring during embryonic life.

⇨ MC sites of coronary fistulae are:

- RCA (55%)
- LCA (35%)
- Both coronaries (05%)

⇨ These fistulae most commonly terminates in:

- RV (40%)
- RA (26%)
- PA (17%)
- Rare sites are Coronary sinus, SVC, LA and LV.

⇨ These fistulae can cause coronary steal leading to ↓ blood supply beyond the connection site.

⇨ The murmur of the coronary fistula is a soft CM with high pitch and superficial nature.

⇨ A fistula draining in the atria may have a CM with loud systolic component due to increased systolic pressure gradient.

⇨ The murmur may be diastolic or a combination of systolic with diastolic murmur if the fistula drains inside the LV.

⇨ Murmur site:

- Left lower border of sternum: Fistula draining inside RV
- Left upper border of sternum: Fistula draining inside LA
- On either side of the lower border of sternum: Fistula draining inside RA.

AORTOPULMONARY WINDOW

⇨ Very rare.

⇨ The CM has a short diastolic part due to a large communication, ↑ PVR, and ↑ PAEDP.

COARCTATION OF AORTA

⇨ Post-ductal: Narrowing distal to left subclavian artery origin and ductus origin.

⇨ Pre-ductal: Diffusely narrowed arch and ascending aorta.

⇨ SBP in arms > legs.

⇨ DBP are similar.

⇨ Suprasternal systolic thrill.

⇨ Ejection systolic murmur along the left border of the sternum and back.

⇨ CM at the interscapular and infrascapular regions due to collateral formation.

⇨ Associated bicuspid aortic valve may produce an ejection click.

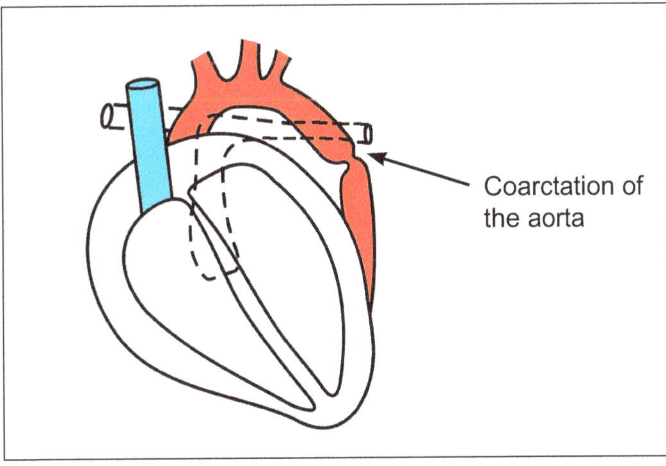

Fig. 17.6

References

- Journal of Medicine and Life Vol. 5, Issue 1, January-March 2012, pp.39-46 ; Continuous murmur - the auscultatory expression of a variety of pathological conditions by Ginghină C, Năstase O A, Ghiorghiu I, Egher L, Carol Davila.
- Clinical methods in cardiology by B Soma Raju.
- JIACM 2011; 12(3):216-20; Approach to a Patient with a Continuous Cardiac Murmur by Prashant Makhija, Sandeep Thakur, Diki Palmu Theengh, Pushpa Yadav, Vivek Arya, AK Agarwal.
- Neoreviews. 2018 July ; 19(7): e394–e402. doi:10.1542/neo.19-7-e394; Diagnosis and Management of Patent Ductus Arteriosus by Maria Gillam-Krakauer and Jeff Reese.
- PERLOFF'S Clinical Recognition of Congenital Heart Disease, Sixth Edition by Joseph K. Perloff; Chapter 20 Patent Ductus Arteriosus Aortopulmonary Window.
- Acta Cardiol Sin 2006;22:96101; Sinus of Valsalva Aneurysm with Rupturing into the Right Atrium A Case Report and Review of the Literature by Chao-Chien Chang, Chih-Hui Chin, Meng-Ling Chen, Thay-Hsiung Chen and Hung-Shun Lo.
- Parashar NK, Bhasin D, Marotrao PS, Farooqui FA, Verma SK, Saxena A. Ruptured sinus of valsalva aneurysm: Clinical case presentation and management. J Pract Cardiovasc Sci 2017;3:109-14.
- Netherlands Heart Journal, Volume 18, Number 4, April 2010; Rupture of right coronary sinus of Valsalva aneurysm into right ventricle by M.C. Post, R.L. Braam, B.E. Groenemeijer, D. Nicastia, B.J. Rensing, M.A. Schepens.
- Ranjan M, Prabhu H, Suresh P. Coronary Cameral Fistulae a Scarce Entity. Adv Card Res 1(1)- 2018. ACR.MS.ID.000101. DOI: 10.32474/ACR.2018.01.000101.
- H H Ho, C W Cheung, M H Jim, L Lam; Heart. 2005 Dec; 91(12): 1540. doi: 10.1136/hrt.2005.064287 PMCID: PMC1769220; Coronary–cameral fistula.
- Cardiol Clin - (2015) - http://dx.doi.org/10.1016/j.ccl.2015.07.011;Coarctation of the Aorta Strategies for Improving Outcomes Lan Nguyen , Stephen C. Cook.
- Manual of practical medicine by R Alagappan;4th edition,Page 138; Coarctation of the aorta.

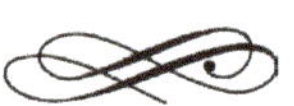

www.ingramcontent.com/pod-product-compliance
Ingram Content Group UK Ltd.
Pitfield, Milton Keynes, MK11 3LW, UK
UKHW061954290726
14090UKWH00021B/1221